ELIMINATING GENDER-BASED VIOLENCE

T0172912

While promoting access to resources and systems of support for those affected by gender-based violence is absolutely crucial, this new book focuses attention on the important question of how communities can take action to prevent violence and abuse.

Using examples of current research and practice, the book explores the actions that can be taken in individual sectors of society, our schools, faith communities, campuses, on our streets and using new popular technologies. The contributors draw on global examples to highlight the importance of learning from the study of the interaction between socio-political contexts and effective policies and strategies to address gender-based violence. Chapters take up the challenge of exploring the construction of effective programmes that address cognitive, affective and behavioural domains. They discuss what people know, how they feel and how they behave, and include the important challenge of how to engage men in working towards the elimination of gender-based violence, offering positive messages which build on men's values and predisposition to act in a positive manner. Importantly, such strategies place the responsibility for preventing gender-based violence on the society as a whole rather than on vulnerable individuals.

This book is essential reading for anyone interested in gender studies, women's studies, social work, sociology, law and health studies. Its unique approach focuses on the achievement of prevention at the earliest possible stage and examines the issue through a society-wide, but community-focused lens.

Ann Taket is Professor of Health and Social Exclusion and director of the Centre for Health through Action on Social Exclusion (CHASE) in the School of Health and Social Development, Deakin University, Australia.

Beth R. Crisp is Professor of Social Work in the School of Health and Social Development, Deakin University, Australia.

ELIMINATING GENDER-BASED VIOLENCE

Edited by Ann Taket and Beth R. Crisp

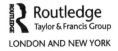

LONDON AND NEW YORK

First published 2018
by Routledge
2 Park Square, Milton Park, Abingdon, Oxon OX14 4RN

and by Routledge
711 Third Avenue, New York, NY 10017

Routledge is an imprint of the Taylor & Francis Group, an informa business

British Library Cataloguing-in-Publication Data
A catalogue record for this book is available from the British Library

Library of Congress Cataloging-in-Publication Data
Names: Taket, A. R. (Ann R.), author. | Crisp, Beth R., author.
Title: Eliminating gender based violence / Ann Taket and Beth R. Crisp.
Description: 1st Edition. | New York: Routledge, 2018. | Includes bibliographical references and index.
Identifiers: LCCN 2017015602| ISBN 9781138924338 (hardback) | ISBN 9781138924345 (pbk.) | ISBN 9781315684437 (ebook)
Subjects: LCSH: Women–Violence against–Prevention.
Classification: LCC HV6250.4.W65 T347 2018 | DDC 362.88/ 16082–dc23LC record available at https://lccn.loc.gov/2017015602

ISBN: 978-1-138-92433-8 (hbk)
ISBN: 978-1-138-92434-5 (pbk)
ISBN: 978-1-315-68443-7 (ebk)

Typeset in Bembo
by Sunrise Setting Ltd, Paignton, UK
Printed and bound by CPI Group (UK) Ltd, Croydon, CR0 4YY

To all those who dare to believe, and dare to act, to eliminate gender-based violence, and to other human rights defenders everywhere.

CONTENTS

ILLUSTRATIONS

Figures

Tables

CONTRIBUTORS

Christine Barter is a Reader in Young People and Violence Prevention in the Connect Centre for International Research on New Approaches to Prevent Violence and Harm, University of Central Lancashire, UK.

Erica Bowen is Professor of Prevention of Violence and Abuse, in the Institute of Health and Society, University of Worcester, UK.

Laura Coady is a Research Assistant in the School of Health and Social Development, Deakin University, Australia.

Beth R. Crisp is Professor of Social Work in the School of Health and Social Development, Deakin University, Australia.

Suzanne Dyson is Associate Professor in the School of Psychology and Public Health, La Trobe University, Australia.

Debbie Ollis is Associate Professor of Education (Health and Physical Education) in the School of Education, Deakin University, Australia.

Cathy Plourde works in publishing, arts, creativity and social innovation from a base in Providence, Rhode Island, US.

Clara Porter is Director of Prevention Action Change, a violence prevention and response organisation in Portland, Maine, US.

Emma Sorbring is Professor of Child and Youth Studies at the Centre for Child and Youth Studies, University West, Sweden.

Ann Taket is Professor of Health and Social Exclusion and director of the Centre for Health through Action on Social Exclusion (CHASE) in the School of Health and Social Development, Deakin University, Australia.

Lynne Marie Wanamaker is Deputy Director at Safe Passage, a domestic violence services organisation in Northampton, Massachusetts, US.

PREFACE

Gender-based violence harms women, families, communities and society in every country and region across the globe. In approaching this book we wanted to focus our attention on the growing evidence base from research and practice around the world that illuminates some effective strategies which can be put in place to work towards the elimination of gender-based violence. At the outset we want to recognise that although resources, services and systems to respond to incidents of violence and abuse which have occurred are vitally important, they are only ever going to be part of the answer if our goal is eliminating gender-based violence. So our main focus in this book is on what is called primary prevention in the public health literature, while recognising, however, that the boundaries between primary and secondary/tertiary prevention can be very indistinct. The book focuses on the achievement of prevention at the earliest possible stage.

Elimination of gender-based violence demands action at all levels and in all sectors of society. Education, workplaces, local government, health and community services as well as residential and cultural communities, all have a part to play. While commitment and leadership at the highest level globally, regionally and nationally are important, so are the actions taken by each and every one of us in the settings of our everyday lives. As various contributions in the book identify, advocacy by local and international non-governmental organisations is vital, as are international and more local feminist movements. The use of intersectional approaches is of particular importance. Tackling other sources of discrimination based on race, class, dis/ability, sexuality, gender identity, ethnicity, religion and culture are also crucial, and there are synergistic benefits to be gained from joint work and endeavours between social movements.

Recent decades have seen growing political consensus about the need for action on gender-based violence. Against this we also see signs of backlash at various levels, most recently and most notably in actions led by the presidents of Russia and the

US which have shown scant disregard for the human rights of women. However, importantly, there is also growing resistance to such backlash, as the final chapter in the book illustrates. We hope this book will stimulate in its readers a sense of the possibilities for action, and reassure them that the goal of elimination of gender-based violence, while requiring considerable and sustained action and change, is an achievable one.

ACKNOWLEDGEMENTS

Funding for the evaluation of *Baby Makes 3* in the Great South Coast that is discussed in Chapter 2 and the evaluation of the Hume regional strategy for preventing violence against women and children that is discussed in Chapter 11 was provided by the Department of Justice and Regulation, Victoria, Australia, as a part of its Reducing Violence against Women and their Children Grants Programme.

ACRONYMS

AAA	Assess, Acknowledge, Act, Sexual Assault Resistance Programme
ACARA	Australian Curriculum and Assessment Authority
ADV	adolescent dating violence
AIDS	acquired immune deficiency syndrome
BM3	*Baby Makes 3*
BMA	British Medical Association
BRR	*Building Respectful Relationships: stepping out against gender-based violence*
CAADA	Co-ordinated Action against Domestic Abuse, UK, now SafeLives
CALCASA	California Coalition against Sexual Assault, US
CAW	Commission on the Advancement of Women
CDC	Centers for Disease Control and Prevention, US
CEDAW	Convention on the Elimination of All Forms of Discrimination against Women
CESCR	Committee on Social, Economic and Cultural Rights
CIDA	Canadian International Development Agency
CRE	couples' relationship education
CSP	*Campus Safety Project*
DOV	Decade to Overcome Violence
DOVE	Doctors Opposing Violence Everywhere, Canada
DV/SA	Domestic violence/sexual assault
ESD	empowerment self-defence
EU	European Union
FGM	female genital mutilation
FRA	European Union Agency for Fundamental Rights
FVPF	Family Violence Prevention Fund, US
GBV	gender-based violence

GDC	General Dental Council, UK
GMC	General Medical Council, UK
HIV	human immunodeficiency virus infection
ICCPR	International Covenant on Civil and Political Rights
ICESCR	International Covenant on Economic, Social and Cultural Rights
IDB	Inter-American Development Bank
IIRR	International Institute of Rural Reconstruction
ILO	International Labour Organization
IMAGE	Intervention with Microfinance for AIDS and Gender Equity
IOM	Institute of Medicine, US
IPPF	International Planned Parenthood Federation
IPV	intimate partner violence
IPVA	interpersonal violence and abuse
IRIS	Identification and Referral to Improve Safety, UK
LGBTIQ	lesbian, gay, bisexual, transgender, intersex and queer
NCAS	National Community Attitudes towards Violence against Women Survey, Australia
NGO	non-governmental organisation
NHS	National Health Service, UK
NICE	National Institute for Health and Care Excellence, UK
NISVS	National Intimate Partner and Sexual Violence Survey, US
NSW	New South Wales, Australia
NWMAF	National Women's Martial Arts Federation, US
OVW	USDOJ Office on Violence against Women
PSHE	personal social and health education
RACGP	Royal Australian College of General Practitioners
RCGP	Royal College of General Practitioners, UK
RCT	randomised controlled trial
RREiS	*Respectful Relationships Education in Schools*
RSE	relationship and sex education
SA	South Australia
SAFFI	South African Faith and Family Institute
SDG	Sustainable Development Goals
SG	serious game
SGBV	sexual and gender-based violence
Sida	Swedish International Development Cooperation Agency
STEM	science, technology, engineering and mathematics
STIR	*Safeguarding Teenage Intimate Relationships*
TAFE	Technical and Further Education, Australia
UK	United Kingdom
UN	United Nations
UNDP	United Nations Development Programme
UN-HABITAT	United Nations Human Settlements Programme
US	United States

USC	United States Congress
USDOE OCR	United States Department of Education Office for Civil Rights
USDOJ	United States Department of Justice
USM	University of Southern Maine, US
VAWA	Violence Against Women Act, 1994, US
WCC	World Council of Churches
WHA	World Health Assembly
WHO	World Health Organization
YPP	*Young Parenthood Program*, US

1

FRAMING THE ISSUES

Ann Taket and Beth R. Crisp

Introduction

Gender-based violence is a significant public health and social welfare problem, as well as a fundamental violation of women's human rights. It is rooted in gender inequalities and reinforces them. Gender-based violence harms women, families, communities and society. It is a major societal issue in every country and region across the globe, with enormous health, economic and social consequences for women, in the short, medium and long term. It also has significant consequences for any children involved in the relationships affected by intimate partner violence, again in the short, medium and long term, accompanied by increased risks of involvement in abusive relationships in the future. Societal costs, in terms of the service responses to health consequences as well as the economic cost in lost production, etc., are also extremely large.

There is a growing political consensus internationally about the need for action on gender-based violence. In 2008, the United Nations Secretary-General Ban Ki-Moon issued a global call to action to end violence against women, by launching the UNiTE to End Violence against Women campaign. The campaign aims to raise public awareness and increase political will and resources for preventing and ending all forms of violence against women and girls in all parts of the world. In March 2013, the agreed conclusions of the 57th session of the Commission on the Status of Women emphasised the importance both of addressing structural and underlying causes and risk factors in order to prevent violence against women and girls, and of strengthening multi-sectoral services, programmes and responses for victims and survivors (Economic and Social Council 2013).

The variation in the prevalence of violence seen within and between communities, countries and regions highlights that violence is not inevitable, and that it can be prevented (Conway et al. 2013). Knowledge about the factors that explain the global variation is growing and evidence is accumulating on promising approaches to the reduction of gender-based violence. This evidence highlights the need to address the economic and socio-cultural factors that foster a culture of violence against women and the importance of promoting equal and respectful relations between men and women. Challenging social norms that support male authority and control over women, and sanction or condone violence against them, is also important, involving promoting non-violent social norms. Reforming discriminatory family law, strengthening women's economic and legal rights, and eliminating gender inequalities in access to formal waged employment and secondary education are all important areas for action. Challenges to sexism, racism, homophobia, transphobia and other types of discrimination based on personal characteristics are all required for a comprehensive approach to preventing gender-based violence.

To respond to the challenge posed by gender-based violence, and in order to ensure that its impacts are progressively reduced, each generation requires a society-wide approach. The elimination of violence occurs incrementally rather than with eradication all at once (Gilligan 2001). Hence, actions taken in settings such as education, workplaces, local government, health and community services, and in sports, as well as in residential and cultural communities, all contribute to society-wide efforts. However, unfortunately the emphasis of many such efforts has been only on limiting the impact of gender-based violence once it has occurred rather than on seeking to prevent it in the first place (for example, Day et al. 2009; Laing et al. 2013), or on minimising it as the action of an individual rather than a consequence of societal conditions and expectations:

> It is therefore necessary to dispel the myth that acts of violence against women are simply unfortunate instances of individual men momentarily losing control. On the contrary, such acts are most often the end of a mindset congruent with the rules of patriarchal power, in which the perpetrator views the woman not as a person . . . but as an 'object to be manipulated'.
>
> (Filemoni-Tofaeono and Johnson 2006: 11)

While promoting access to resources and systems of support for those affected by gender-based violence is absolutely crucial, this book focuses attention on the important question of how communities can take action to prevent violence and abuse. Using current research and practice, it explores actions that can be taken in different sectors of society. We draw on research and developing practice across the globe, highlighting the importance of learning from nuanced study of the interaction between socio-political context and effective policies and strategies to address gender-based violence. Chapters take up the challenge of exploring the construction of effective programmes that address cognitive, affective and behavioural domains – what people think, how they feel and how they behave – including the important challenge of how to engage men in working towards the elimination of gender-based violence, and offering positive messages which build on men's values and predisposition to act in a positive manner. Importantly, such strategies place the responsibility for preventing gender-based violence on the society as a whole rather than on vulnerable individuals.

This chapter begins by introducing the theoretical frameworks that underlie our understanding of gender-based violence, including: the socio-ecological model; Hagemann-White et al.'s (2010) multi-level model of factors at play in the perpetration of violence against women and children and sexual orientation violence; intersectionality; and the multi-systems life-course perspective. As should be clear from the frameworks included, the chapter draws on perspectives from a variety of different disciplines. It will then discuss the society-wide approach required to prevent gender-based violence, examining examples of research and practice drawn from around the globe. This will offer a chance to ensure that the coverage in the book as a whole is truly global, by including more detailed sections on gaps that remain uncovered by Chapters 2 to 11. The chapter will end by introducing the remaining chapters in the book, in the context of both the theoretical frameworks introduced and society-wide approaches.

Gender-based violence: understanding the causes

> Gendered violence does not exist in isolation, and is intertwined with other forms of power, privilege and social exclusion.
>
> *(Shahrokh 2015: 1)*

The above quote succinctly summarises the fundamental stance taken in this volume that gender-based violence does not occur in a vacuum, and that attempts to eliminate gender-based violence without taking into account issues of power, privilege and social exclusion are fanciful and unrealistic. Furthermore, as Article 1 of the United Nations (UN) *Declaration on the Elimination of Violence against Women* recognises, there is a multitude of ways in which gender-based violence occurs and the resulting impacts of such violence:

> any act of gender based violence that results in, or is likely to result in, physical, sexual or psychological harm or suffering to women, including threats of such acts, coercion, or arbitrary deprivation of liberty, whether occurring in public or in private life.
>
> *(UN 1993: Article 1)*

We have adopted this definition for a number of reasons: first of all it subsumes different types of abuse into the single term violence, including unethical and immoral behaviours which may not be illegal in addition to those which are illegal (Messina-Dysert 2015). Second, it emphasises not only enacted violence, but also threats of violence and forms of 'entertainment' which result in 'the annihilation of connectivity, the dulling and erasure of human relationality through objectivication' (Cooper-White 1995: 18). Third, it explicitly refers to both public and private domains, which is particularly important as it is vital that violence and abuse is not excused on the grounds of it happening in the domain of the private.

It is also important that this definition is understood as including anyone who identifies as female. Violence is experienced by people whose experience and/or identity does not conform to binary definitions of sex and gender, and while this book does not explicitly discuss preventing violence against transgender, gender diverse and intersex people, it should be noted that such violence shares some similar drivers to violence against women (particularly rigid, binary and hierarchical constructions of gender, sex and sexuality).

Finally, although the UN definition refers to 'women', experiences of gender-based violence are not confined to adults but can occur at any age, although the ways in which it occurs can vary for infants, children, adolescents, adults and elderly persons (Filemoni-Tofaeono and Johnson 2006).

The roots of the current understanding of factors underlying gender-based violence lie in the ecological models proposed to link behavioural analysis that focuses on the individual in their local setting and the analysis of whole societies. One of the best known is Bronfenbrenner's Ecological Framework for Human Development (Bronfenbrenner 1979, 2005). Ecological approaches were applied to understandings of child abuse and neglect (Belsky 1980) and later to domestic violence (for example, Carlson 1984; Dutton 1988; Edleson and Tolman 1992). In 1998, Heise built on these earlier efforts to provide an integrated ecological approach to gender-based violence (Heise 1998). This was taken up in the 2002 *World Report on Violence and Health* (Krug et al. 2002), which included an ecological model of violence, reinforcing the connections between causation and prevention of all different types of violence. This is discussed further below.

The socio-ecological model

The socio-ecological model places the individual in the centre of their world, surrounded in turn by their interpersonal, community, societal and global environments. The interpersonal includes family (defined by biology, adoption, choice) and friends, whereas community refers to the different settings of everyday life, including schools, workplaces, and various different settings for leisure and service use. At a societal level, social relations are affected by social and economic policy as well as by the media. In the wake of increasing globalisation and internationalisation, to capture the influence of the work of international organisations such as the UN and its various bodies, as well as bi- and multi-lateral factors such as trade, development aid and so on, a global level has been added to the original model to represent supranational factors.

Gender-based violence occurs in interpersonal, community, societal and global contexts, and can impact on individuals, groups and communities, and their relationships with each other and more generally with humanity. Hence, a range of responses is required in both responding to violence which has occurred and preventing further violence from eventuating. For example, the Prevention Institute's

Spectrum of Prevention distinguishes six levels at which prevention efforts operate, ranging from micro-level approaches aimed at raising awareness and changing violence-related attitudes among individuals to macro-level strategies that attempt to shift broader social norms and enact policy supporting violence-free societies (Davis et al. 2006).

Perhaps one of the most highly detailed multi-level ecological models is that developed for the European Commission as part of a feasibility study to assess the possibilities, opportunities and needs to standardise national legislation on gender violence and violence against children. Hagemann-White et al. (2010, n.d.) have produced an interactive model of the factors at play in violence against women and children and sexual orientation violence. Based on the existing body of research into perpetration, they distinguish nine different categories of violence, which could be influenced by policy or practical intervention, and show the factors implicated in each of them (see Table 1.1). Table 1.2 summarises the main factors that have been identified as being associated with gender-based violence at macro- (society), meso- (institutions, agencies, social environments), micro- (face-to-face social groups) and ontogenetic (individual life history) levels.

TABLE 1.1 Nine categories/types of violence

1 Rape/sexual coercion
2 Partner violence/stalking
3 Sexual harassment
4 Trafficking
5 Harmful traditional practices
6 Child abuse and neglect
7 Child sexual abuse
8 Child sexual exploitation
9 Violence based on sexual orientation

Source: Compiled from Hagemann-White et al. (n.d.).

TABLE 1.2 Factors conducive to violence against women, violence against children and sexual orientation violence, by four levels

Ontogenetic	Micro	Meso	Macro
Poor parenting	Stereotypes	Failed sanctions	Devaluing women
Early trauma	Obedience code	Honour codes	Masculinity
Emotions	Family stressors	Hate groups	Children's status
Cognitions	Rewards	Entitlement	Media violence
Masculine self	Opportunity	Discrimination	Impunity
Depersonalised sex	Peer approval	Poverty pockets	
Stimulus abuse			

Source: Compiled from Hagemann-White et al. (n.d.).

For each of the nine types of violence distinguished, the different factors at each of the levels associated with them are identified, together with whether the influence is weak, moderate or strong (according to the available evidence); this is the perpetration perspective. The factor perspective summarises the size of the effect of each factor on the nine different types of violence. A separate page gives access to the path models for different forms of violence. For each form of violence the models show the particular factors and pathways by which they are influenced; this enables interactions between the different factors to be seen, which are different for each form of violence.

Protective factors and interventions are also shown. The authors caution that the models are a tool for strategic thinking, and do not provide any straightforward recommendations, and furthermore are limited by the availability of research evidence. In particular they emphasise that although much of the research is concentrated at the individual level, this should not be seen as reducing the importance of the other levels, as they summarise:

> The fact that ontogenetic factors have been more extensively studied and more frequently measured empirically should not be taken to mean that the primary causal influences are to be found within the individual's history and personality. For the vast majority of individuals, these factors will only lead to violent behaviour when there is a conducive context permitting or encouraging this outcome.
>
> *(Hagemann-White et al. 2010: 78)*

Intersectionality

Intersectionality is useful to further deepen understanding of gender-based violence. Intersectionality (or intersectional theory) is a term first coined in 1989 by Crenshaw (1989, 1991). It is the study of overlapping or intersecting social identities and related systems of oppression, domination or discrimination. Intersectionality posits that multiple identities intersect to create a whole that is different from the component identities. These identities that can intersect include gender, race, social class, ethnicity, nationality, sexual orientation, religion, age, and different types of dis/ability in both physical and mental domains. These aspects of identity are not 'unitary, mutually exclusive entities, but rather . . . reciprocally constructing phenomena' (Collins 2015: 2). As Crenshaw (1991) discusses, the violence that women experience depends on their positionality in relation to all the other dimensions of their identities in interaction. Figure 1.1 shows these intersectional characteristics operating across all the different levels in the socio-ecological model.

Preventing gender-based violence requires recognising intersectional interactions and responding to them when designing interventions across the whole spectrum of responses required to gender-based violence, from primary prevention through to services to respond to the needs of those who experience gender-based violence as well as of those who perpetrate it. Intersectional analysis is essential if we are to

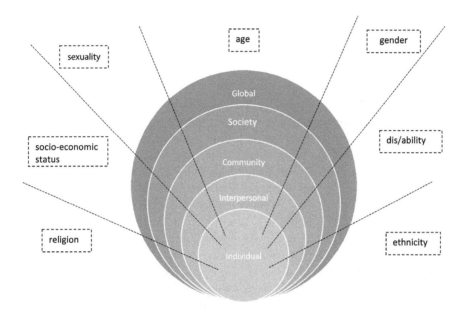

FIGURE 1.1 Modified socio-ecological model and intersectional characteristics

understand what works for who, how and where. The implications of intersectional analysis for primary prevention are being increasingly explored. Guedes et al. (2016: 1) present a global review of intersections of violence against women and violence against children, and conclude that 'consolidating efforts to address shared risk factors may help prevent both forms of violence'; the specific opportunities they identify include primary prevention (school-based strategies, parenting programmes) and early intervention. Drawing on case study research addressing sexual and gender-based violence in Egypt, India, Kenya, Sierra Leone, South Africa and Uganda, Shahrokh (2015) demonstrates how intersectional analysis has supported gender-justice movements, in particular through supporting cross-movement alliance building.

One area where intersectional analysis has proved very useful is in the scrutiny of policy to identify how policies can be made more inclusive and effective. Strid et al. (2013) examined British policy on violence against women from 2001 to 2011. They examined the visibility of multiple inequalities and their intersections, arguing that until equality is reached, visibility is a strategic method, enabling special measures that address particular intersections. The analysis distinguishes three different levels of visibility: the naming of inequalities; the intersections in practice between inequalities and how they work structurally through intersecting fields of violence, and relevant policy domains; and the inclusion of the voices of minoritised women in defining the structural intersections in policy outcomes. In terms of the three specific policy fields, they consider domestic violence, sexual violence and forced marriage, and find that simple naming of inequality grounds (domestic violence policy) is the weakest form of visibility and inclusion, while the inclusion of the voices of minoritised women is the strongest form of visibility and inclusion (forced marriage policy). A final important point that Strid et al. (2013) emphasise is the need to ensure that gender does not become invisible, with the attendant risk that specific forms of violence become culturalised, ethnicised or racialised rather than gendered.

Lombardo and Agustin (2016: 371) present an analysis of a selection of European Union policies on gender-based violence during the period 2000 to 2014, finding, 'with respect to domestic violence . . . little evidence of an awareness of intersections between gender and other inequalities in EU policy framework', identifying that much remains to be done in terms of improving the overall quality of policies.

At a totally different level of analysis, White and Peretz (2010: 403) use an intersectional analysis of Black masculinities to explore how negative emotions raised by becoming aware of injustice to a woman were transformed by organisational activities of becoming active in the pro-feminist movement into positive emotions, by fostering 'new raced-gendered feeling rules regarding emotion that challenge hegemonic masculinity generally and Black hegemonic masculinities, in particular'. Their analysis has particularly important messages for the challenge of engaging men in preventing gender-based violence, which this chapter returns to later.

The multi-systems life-course perspective

The final theoretical approach to understanding gender-based violence introduced in this chapter is the multi-system life-course perspective which is a

> dynamic, complex and holistic approach that considers the significance of biological, psychological, social, political, cultural, and historical realities over time and the influences that such factors have on the development of the trajectory or path of any organism (individuals, families, groups, communities, organizations, nations, etc.)
>
> *(Murphy-Erby et al. 2010: 677)*

The key feature of this approach is its focus on dynamics. While Murphy-Erby et al. (2010) explore the implications of the approach for social work practice and a graduate social work curriculum, the approach has found much more frequent use in research into trajectories of victimhood/survivorship and perpetration. So, for example, Macmillan (2001) looked at victimisation over the life course, examining life-course development in terms of psychological distress and well-being, involvement in crime and deviance, and educational and socio-economic attainment; Draucker and Martsolf (2010) identified six different life-course typologies of individuals who had been exposed to sexual violence; Jennings and Reingle (2012) carried out a narrative meta-review to describe the number and shape of violence, aggression and delinquency trajectories; and finally, Shah et al. (2016) explore disabled women's experience of gender-based violence and support, importantly including examples of impairment-specific violence that non-disabled women do not experience.

Looking specifically at opportunities for prevention, Etherington and Baker (2016) explore links between boys' victimisation and adult perpetration of intimate partner violence. The exploration is limited to examination of programmes with supportive evidence from randomised controlled trials and concentrated mainly on individual level, and on secondary and tertiary prevention.

A society-wide approach to primary prevention

> Patriarchy is not new. It is a system created and maintained by men of faith and politics who hold the levers of economic, cultural, and political power and who confuse strength and masculinity with domination and brutality. Patriarchy must be replaced by a system in which equal human rights and non-violence are promoted and accepted. This will happen if we embrace the kind of love and mutual respect exemplified and preached by the founders of the world's great religions, and through the persistent efforts of those who speak out and work for a more equal and less violent world. Equal human dignity is a human right, as codified in many global treaties. It is my hope that political and religious leaders will step forward and use their influence to communicate clearly that violence against women and girls must stop, that we are failing our societies, and that the time for leadership is now.
>
> *(Carter 2015: e41)*

In 2015, the medical journal *The Lancet* published a landmark series of review articles on violence against women and girls (Ellsberg et al. 2015; Garcia-Moreno et al. 2015a, 2015b; Jewkes et al. 2015; Michau et al. 2015), together with three short comments; the quotation that heads this section is taken from one of these. This series was significant for a number of reasons, most importantly that it marked an important acknowledgement that gender inequality is a root driver of gender-based violence, and that, as a consequence, eliminating gender-based violence requires nothing less than a society-wide systemic approach, at multiple levels, to address the economic, political and social structures that subordinate women, based on an intersectional analysis that recognises the other factors that are at play. Currently, there is no country in the world where such an approach fully exists; instead, we see countries with implementation in only some of the different areas where action is required. However, what can be seen around the globe is a growing body of evidence and promising practice that illuminates the way forward.

The elimination of gender-based violence is central to equitable and sustainable development. Ensuring that programming in all sectors is gender transformative is essential. It is also important to recognise that programmes that address gender norms, as drivers of men's violence against women, also address drivers of men's violence against men and of men's violence against children (Garcia-Moreno et al. 2015b). Fleming et al. (2015) explore this in detail for men's violence against women and men's violence against men, and argue for more interdisciplinary and multi-sectoral action to tackle all types of violence through addressing their root causes. Based on empirical research among women's anti-war organisations world-wide, Cockburn (2010, 2012) demonstrates that patriarchal gender relations are intersectional with economic and ethno-national power relations in perpetuating a tendency to armed conflict in human societies.

Continued activism by autonomous women's movements is important. Htun and Weldon (2012) demonstrated in their analysis of policy changes in seventy countries over the period 1975 to 2005 that the main driver of progressive governments' action on gender-based violence was the presence of such autonomous movements.

At the international level, the UN has made significant progress towards gender equality through such agreements as the *Beijing Declaration and Platform for Action* and the *Convention on the Elimination of All Forms of Discrimination against Women* (CEDAW). In 2010, a new UN entity was created, UN Women, bringing together relevant parts of the UN system which focused on gender equality and women's empowerment. The three main roles of UN Women are: to support inter-governmental bodies, such as the Commission on the Status of Women, in their formulation of policies, global standards and norms; to help Member States to implement these standards, standing ready to provide suitable technical and financial support to those countries that request it, and to forge effective partnerships with civil society; and to lead and coordinate the UN system's work on gender equality as well as promote accountability, including through regular monitoring of system-wide progress (UN Women n.d.). As an example, just one of the areas in which they are working, gender mainstreaming, is explored in the next section.

After considering gender mainstreaming, the chapter moves on to consider examples of two more areas of work that are essential to eliminating gender-based violence. The first of these covers initiatives aimed at economic empowerment, which can be regarded as examples of specific mechanisms for gender mainstreaming in employment/economic sectors. This is one of the areas where specific programmes of work have been subject to very rigorous evaluation using randomised control trials. Following that, a section on the *SASA!* programme considers an example of a community mobilisation approach that has been subject to a quite extensive programme of research involving a cluster randomised controlled trial with a nested qualitative study. A further section introduces some of the challenges remaining, before the final one introduces the remainder of the chapters in the book.

Gender mainstreaming

Gender mainstreaming is an interesting case of a strategy that has been globally diffused as a result of the processes associated with globalisation (True and Mintrom 2001). In their study of the proliferation of state bureaucracies for gender mainstreaming, True and Mintrom understand it as 'efforts to scrutinize and reinvent processes of policy formulation and implementation across all issue areas to address and rectify persistent and emerging disparities between men and women' (2001: 28).

Noting that a decision was made at the 1975 UN International Women's Year conference that all governments should establish agencies dedicated to promoting gender equality, they carried out an event history analysis of 157 nation states from 1975 to 1998, identifying 100 such agencies in place by 1997. Their analysis discovered that the transnational networking of non-state actors (for example, non-government organisations) has been the primary force driving the diffusion, in particular women's international non-governmental organisations, the transnational feminist movement and the United Nations.

Since the Fourth UN World Women's Conference in 1995, gender mainstreaming has been endorsed by nearly every important international organisation (Hafner-Burton and Pollack 2002). Gender mainstreaming was defined in the Beijing Platform for Action as applying 'a gender perspective in all policies and programmes so that, before decisions are taken, an analysis is made of the effects on women and men, respectively' (Fourth World Conference on Women 1995: paragraph 189). The first efforts to implement mainstreaming occurred inside the UN Development Programme and in other multi-lateral development organisations such as the International Labour Organisation (ILO) and the World Bank (Razavi and Miller 1995).

In the very brief discussion offered here, it should be acknowledged there is insufficient space to address the literature on gender mainstreaming as a contested concept (see for example the 2005 special issue of *Social Politics* introduced by Walby 2005); instead the discussion concentrates on the practice of gender mainstreaming as a process to promote gender equality, thereby tackling one of the root drivers of gender-based violence.

Various tools, checklists, manuals and handbooks have been produced to aid implementation: development in environment and energy (UNDP 2007), in local government (for example UN-HABITAT 2008), in development programming (for example UN Women 2014), in the health sector (for example WHO 2011), and for international development organisations (Gilles 2015); this last is particularly useful since it offers an excellent overview of many different tools for use within the organisational setting, not just in development organisations. UN Women has a downloadable repository of resources and tools with hotlinks, covering what has been produced by various agencies in the UN system (UN Women n.d.).

Empirical research into the effectiveness of gender mainstreaming in implementation remains limited. There have been a number of studies of international organisations/bodies and their progress with gender mainstreaming. Pollack and Hafner-Burton (2000) studied gender mainstreaming in the European Union (EU) by examining implementation in five areas of EU policy: structural funds, employment, development, competition, and science, research and development. They found that progress has been quite variable across issue areas, reflecting the considerable variation in political opportunities, mobilising structure and dominant frames or discourses characterising each of the responsible Directorates General. They also identified that advocates of gender mainstreaming have been strategic and sophisticated in framing gender mainstreaming as an efficient means whereby officials in a broad range of areas can achieve their goals. They identified achievement of main-streaming goals in four of the five areas, but note three distinct points of critique: concern about the abandonment of positive actions on behalf of women; limited nature of outcomes, administrative procedures and 'soft law' proclamations, failing to create legally enforceable rights; and finally the dominance of an integration-ist approach, whereby a gender perspective is introduced into existing processes, rather than an agenda-setting approach involving a fundamental re-thinking of policy goals from a gender perspective. Another analysis of gender mainstreaming in Europe is provided by Rees (2005), who examined to what extent the tools associ-ated with different principles underlying mainstreaming have been introduced in the countries of the EU (or even parts of countries). At this different level she found a highly uneven level of implementation.

Hafner-Burton and Pollack (2002) examined implementation in two interna-tional organisations, the United Nations Development Programme (UNDP) and the World Bank. Their analysis concluded that the relatively rapid acceptance of gender mainstreaming during the 1980s and 1990s was due to the political oppor-tunities surrounding the UNDP as well as the dominant discourse in that agency. The dominant neoliberal discourse in the World Bank combined with relatively scarce elite allies and access points for the arguments for gender mainstreaming put forward by advocates. However, the World Bank did eventually adopt main-streaming as official policy, following a series of studies demonstrating the gains in economic efficiency from investment in women, and has made considerable progress since 1995. In contrast to the UNDP, the World Bank's greater leverage in countries with recipient governments dependent on World Bank funding has resulted in more effective implementation.

Moser (2005) examined the experiences of international development agen-cies in the South, including the work of the Canadian International Development Agency (CIDA), the Swedish International Development Cooperation Agency (Sida), the World Bank, the Inter-American Development Bank (IDB) and the UK government's Department for International Development, and analyses four different stages in gender mainstreaming: embracing the terminology of gender equality and gender mainstreaming; getting a gender mainstreaming policy into place; implementing gender mainstreaming in practice; and finally, evaluating or auditing the practice of gender mainstreaming. Evidence of widespread consensus and achievement in the first two of these stages was found, with less progress in the other two. Moser also concluded that the 'best practices' from the South may provide useful lessons for those confronting problems of gender mainstreaming in the North. This is borne out in some of the work discussed later in the book (for example Chapter 11).

The final two examples considered here are compendiums of promising practice with a strong theoretical base. The first of these dealt with case studies of successful innovation from across Asia and the Pacific, covering sectors as diverse as health, civil and political participation, natural resource management, infrastructure devel-opment and organisational transformation, as well as some programmes specifically around gender-based violence (InterAction-CAW and IIRR 2004). Finally, James-Sebro (2005) explored five international NGOs working in four African countries: World Vision in Ghana; Catholic Relief Services and Lutheran World Relief in Kenya; CARE in Niger; and Heifer Project International in Zambia. This was a study with detailed field research involving nearly nine hundred people in 16 rural communities. Findings included reports of declines in practices such as female genital mutilation (FGM), early and/or forced marriages and opposition to girls' education, as well as improvements in equality in property rights and inheritance. Together women and men also explored new roles in daily chores as well as agriculture. Linking gender equality to poverty, including the poverty of men and of communities, proved to be a catalyst for acceptance in communities. Other examples that exist focus on one component only, on gender equality training or on the use of a particular tool or manual, rather than taking an organisation- or system-wide approach; these are not discussed here.

A remaining challenge for the future is to build in sufficiently robust processes for monitoring and evaluation to continue to build knowledge about promising and effective practice. In an effort to support this process and offer helpful guidance that also recognises the need to take into account intersectional issues, a further publication from UN Women covers inclusive systemic evaluation for gender equality, environments and voices from the margins (Stephens et al. 2017). This has specifically been produced with the Sustainable Development Goals in mind, the strapline for which is 'leaving no one behind'.

Economic empowerment

One relatively frequent component of programmes of gender mainstreaming in the employment/economic sector(s) is schemes for the development of economic empowerment, including provision of microcredit. This is also an area where some specific programmes of work have been subject to very rigorous evaluation using randomised control trials. Evaluations of some of these programmes have directly measured impact on intimate partner violence, while others have examined effects on other aspects of gender-based violence, for example child marriage.

The Intervention with Microfinance for AIDS and Gender Equity (IMAGE), initially trialled in rural South Africa, combined a microfinance programme with participatory training on understanding HIV infection, gender norms, domestic violence and sexuality (Kim et al. 2007). A cluster randomised trial design was used. Outcome measures included experience of intimate partner violence over the previous year and indicators of women's empowerment. Qualitative data about changes occurring within intimate relationships, loan groups and the community were also collected. At the end of two years, the risk of past-year physical or sexual violence by an intimate partner was reduced by more than half and improvements in all indicators of empowerment were observed. The qualitative data found that reductions in violence resulted from a range of responses enabling women to challenge the acceptability of violence, expect and receive better treatment from partners, leave abusive relationships, and raise public awareness about intimate part-ner violence. Kim et al. (2007) concluded that economic and social empowerment of women can contribute to reductions in intimate partner violence. The IMAGE intervention is being scaled up in South Africa and implemented in Tanzania and Peru (Ellsberg et al. 2015).

Two further studies with randomised designs of unconditional cash transfer pro-grammes in Kenya (Haushofer and Shapiro 2013) and Ecuador (Hidrobo et al. 2015) reported significant reductions in rates of intimate partner violence, as well as economic and nutritional benefits to households. Incentives, financial or material, have been found to reduce child marriage in a number of studies. An Ethiopian intervention (Erulkar and Muthengi 2009) combined an economic incentive for girls to remain at school with other forms of support and education/training. This was associated with improvements in school enrolment, age at marriage, repro-ductive health knowledge and contraceptive use. Duflo et al. (2006) reported on a study that evaluated the impact of four HIV/AIDS prevention interventions, implemented in rural Kenyan schools between 2002 and 2005, on limiting teenage childbearing, one of which involved an economic incentive to remain in school, namely a free school uniform; they found that reducing education costs in this way is effective in lowering teenage childbearing and marriage rates. Baird et al. (2011) described a randomised trial in Malawi which compared an unconditional cash transfer with a conditional transfer (conditional on school attendance) and a control group with no transfer. School attendance and achievement was greatest in the conditional group, yet teenage pregnancy and marriage rates were lowest in the unconditional group and highest in the no transfer group. Nanda et al. (2014) described a programme established in 1994 in India that used savings bonds as an incentive to encourage parents not to marry off their daughters before they were aged 18 years. The savings bond was redeemable when the daughter reached 18, only if she was not married. Preliminary findings from continuing assessment indicate that beneficiary girls have higher educational attainment compared with non-beneficiaries. There was no impact on marrying before age 18, but some indi-cation that marriage occurred later (shortly after reaching 18). The authors point to the absence of socially acceptable alternatives to marriage post-18 as being respon-sible (Nanda et al. 2014).

Hansen (2015) studied the effect of a microfinance intervention on psychologi-cal empowerment among women in north Sri Lanka. Psychological empowerment is defined as personal and social capacity for action. The intervention included rel-evant skills training, saving activities, and micro loans to eligible clients. A random sample of women who had participated in the programme for 12–18 months were selected and compared with a matched control group. Women in the interven-tion group showed higher levels of both personal and social capacity compared with the control group. Also, importantly, women who received training showed stronger effects than women who did not, illustrating the importance of training to capacitate women (Hansen 2015). Finally, Al Shami et al. (2016) examined the effect of a specific microcredit institution on Malay Muslim women in an urban area. They carried out a mixed methods study involving a cross-sectional survey of old and new clients (the new clients who had not yet received loans served as a control group) and informal semi-structured interviews with a sample of current clients who had received credit for starting new businesses two years previously. Training of several types is provided before microcredit is received and there are weekly group meetings. The investigators reported that the Malay Muslim women had been empowered, in both social and economic terms at household and community levels, after receiving microcredit. Household decision-making had shifted from being solely a domain of men, to one where women did this jointly with their husbands. Women's movement outside their homes had improved because of the programme, as well as their social status in their communities.

SASA! – a community mobilisation model in Kampala, Uganda

SASA! is a community mobilisation intervention that aims to tackle gender inequality, violence against women and HIV vulnerability for women by changing community attitudes, norms and behaviours (Abramsky et al. 2014). The intervention was designed using the ecological model as a framework (Abramsky et al. 2014) and the stages of change theory underlying individual behaviour change (Abramsky et al. 2016b). The intervention was evaluated using a pair-matched cluster randomised controlled trial in eight communities in Kampala, Uganda (Abramsky et al. 2014, 2016b).

Within each community the aim of the intervention is to promote critical analysis and discussion of power and power inequalities, focusing on the use of power to effect and sustain change at the community level, as well as on how men and women may misuse power and the resulting consequences for intimate relationships and communities (Abramsky et al. 2014). SASA! is an acronym for the four stages in the intervention (Abramsky et al. 2014). The first stage is 'start' – in which community activists, both men and women, are selected and trained along with staff from selected organisations such as police and health care. This group of activists then lead the work through the other three stages. In the second stage, 'awareness', activists stimulate informal activities, encouraging critical thinking about 'power over' women. Four strategies are used: local activism, media and advocacy, communication materials and training. The specifics of what happens in each community is not prescribed, but allowed to develop and evolve in relation to community characteristics and locally generated priorities and needs. In the third stage, 'support', work continues to strengthen the skills of and connection between community members, joining with others to support change. In the fourth stage, 'action', new behaviours are instigated and change celebrated. Each stage builds on the ones before, with an increasing number of individuals and groups involved. The acronym SASA! also very appropriately means 'now' in Kiswahili. SASA! was designed by Raising Voices, a non-profit organisation based in Kampala, and was implemented in Kampala by the Centre for Domestic Violence Prevention (a local civil society organisation), based around the use of the *SASA! Activist Kit for Preventing Violence against Women and HIV* (Michau 2008).

The evaluation of *SASA!* made baseline measurements in cross-sectional community surveys of people aged 18–49 in each of the intervention and control communities, with follow-up measurements four years after intervention implementation (Abramsky et al. 2016b). Outcomes measured included women's past-year experiences of physical and sexual intimate partner violence, emotional aggression, controlling behaviours and fear of partner. At follow-up, all types of intimate partner violence (including severe forms of each) were lower in intervention than in control communities (Abramsky et al. 2016b). Statistically significant effects were observed for continued physical intimate partner violence, sexual intimate partner violence, emotional aggression and fear of partner, as well as for new onset of controlling behaviours. Abramsky et al. (2016b) concluded that community mobilisation is effective in terms of both primary and secondary prevention.

A further analysis of the trial data reported in Abramsky et al. (2016a) examined the mediating role of community-, relationship- and individual-level factors on past-year experience of intimate partner violence (women) and experience of perpetration (men). They found that community-level normative attitudes were the most important mediators of intervention impact on experience and perpetration, while reduced acceptability of intimate partner violence among men was the most important individual-level mediator (Abramsky et al. 2016a).

As well as the trial, a nested qualitative study explored pathways of relationship- and community-level change as a result of *SASA!* (Kyegombe et al. 2014). This involved in-depth interviews carried out at follow-up with 20 women and 20 men from the intervention communities who reported reductions in the levels of violence they had experienced or used in the previous 12 months. As Kyegombe et al. (2014) report, not all participants reported change at either level. At the relationship level participants reported that *SASA!* helped them to explore the benefits of mutually supportive gender roles, improve communication, increase levels of joint decision-making and deal with anger or disagreement in non-violent ways, while at the community level, participants reported that *SASA!* helped foster non-tolerance of violence through reducing the acceptability of violence and increasing individuals' skills, willingness and sense of responsibility to act to prevent intimate partner violence, as well as developing and strengthening community-based structures (Kyegombe et al. 2014). A different part of the qualitative study examined children's exposure to violence (Kyegombe et al. 2015). As well as the sample of community members referred to above, a further 10 community members with children were recruited (since not all the original 40 were living with children), along with 20 community activists and 12 community leaders (in each case split evenly between men and women). Analysis of this qualitative data suggested parenting and discipline practices sometimes also changed – improving parent–child relationships and, for a few parents, resulting in the complete rejection of corporal punishment as a disciplinary method (Kyegombe et al. 2015). Some participants also reported intervening to prevent violence against children.

Taken together, the findings from the *SASA!* trial give strong support for the more widespread adoption of community-level approaches to preventing violence, and indicate that interventions to prevent IPV may also impact on children's exposure to violence and improve parent–child relationships. Furthermore, the findings suggest that interventions to prevent intimate partner violence may also contribute to violence prevention in other areas, specifically against children (Kyegombe et al. 2015).

Introducing the chapters that follow

In the remainder of this book there are nine chapters, Chapters 2 to 11 inclusive, that focus on particular topics, before Chapter 12, the concluding chapter, summarises the key issues identified, presents overall implications for the prevention of gender-based violence and makes recommendations for future work.

Chapter 2 focuses on working with parents and young families. There is an increasing number of programmes that work with parents and young families, including programmes aimed at preventing child abuse and maltreatment, at preventing adolescent problem behaviours (including perpetration of violence and abuse) and at promoting respectful relationships between parents. In this chapter the literature on the effectiveness of these programmes is reviewed, drawing on work carried out around the world, and distinguishing between programmes that target different groups considered 'at risk' in some fashion and those that adopt a more universal approach. A particular focus of the chapter is on recent research from Australia into one particular parenting programme aimed at all first-time parents, *Baby Makes 3*. This programme seeks to assist couples as they transition into parenthood, and demonstrates an extremely promising area of practice.

Chapters 3 to 6 then focus on work with young people, oriented at specific age groups and in specific settings. Chapter 3 looks at healthy and respectful relationships education in schools. Teaching about gender-based violence has always presented challenges for schools. A lack of recognition of gender-based violence, perceived and real opposition, teacher confidence and professional development, and competing curriculum priorities have all been shown to present barriers to effective approaches in schools. Over the past five years a number of school-based pilot projects designed to prevent gender-based violence and build respectful relationships have been trialled in secondary schools in Victoria, Australia. The trials have utilised classroom materials developed in line with the findings of a commissioned report that argued for a new approach to violence prevention. The report's authors argued for a feminist theoretical framework addressing the link between gendered power relations, inequalities and violence against women. This chapter examines how the key elements of 'best practice' recommended in this report worked in reality for schools and one university in the implementation of education about gender-based violence and respectful relationships. By exploring in-service and pre-service teachers' and students' experiences of being involved in these trials, the chapter examines the barriers and enablers to effective practice, including whether the content and approaches in the materials were useful in assisting teachers to teach about gender-based violence. In addition, it explores the potential or otherwise this has for increasing student and teacher understanding of the issues and intended agency to prevent gender-based violence and build respectful relationships.

Chapter 4 focuses on adolescence and explores the use of technology to prevent violence and abuse in romantic relationships. Traditional approaches to the primary prevention of violence and abuse in adolescent romantic relationships (known as dating violence) have adopted didactic classroom-based pedagogic designs. However, there exists compelling evidence that games-based pedagogic approaches can lead to increased knowledge acquisition and retention, and there is an increasing literature documenting the impact of these approaches in mainstream curricula subjects. This chapter provides an overview of the literature in relation to the potential of games-based, and more specifically computer-mediated games-based education, taking as a case study the *Green Acres High* 'serious game', developed by partners in England, Sweden, Belgium and Germany. Preliminary evaluation data support the potential role that technology could play in combating adolescent dating violence, and practical, ethical and safeguarding issues surrounding the development and implementation of such intervention approaches are discussed.

Chapter 5 also focuses on adolescence and covers work on safeguarding in teenage intimate relationships being carried out in the UK, Cyprus, Bulgaria, Italy and Norway. The project contributes to the safeguarding of young people's welfare by raising awareness of this under-researched form of intimate violence; enabling young people's experiences and views to inform policy and practice; and enhancing the development of appropriate prevention and intervention programmes across Europe. The chapter discusses the issues involved in the development of an appropriate, directly accessible, web-based resource and app for young people.

Chapter 6 moves into a slightly older age group by considering campus-based programmes to address sexual assault. Such programmes in the US often struggle to be truly supportive and safe to enable a victim to make a disclosure. This chapter considers an alternative approach involving a university-wide programme to promote healthy relationships and prevent and better respond to sexual assault and harassment, domestic and dating violence, and stalking in the campus community. This programme spurred major policy and protocol changes, law enforcement and conduct board training, and creation of bystander intervention and peer-support initiatives, and resulted in a dramatic increase in crime reporting by students on three campuses.

Chapter 7 examines the potential offered by feminist empowerment self-defence (ESD). Arising from the grassroots feminist movement as an activist response to sexual and gendered violence, ESD has matured into a cogent, comprehensive methodology, including professional standards for ESD instructors and a social justice-informed, survivor-centred ethos. The act of teaching women to fight challenges gender-based social norms around body autonomy and physical power. ESD is a strength-based intervention empowering those at heightened risk for sexual and gendered violence with concrete tools to improve their own circumstances. By defining sexual and gendered violence as a cultural rather than individual problem, ESD encourages social critique and collective action.

Engaging bystanders in violence prevention is the topic of Chapter 8. Changing social norms is a key component in achieving effective prevention of violence, and the potentially important role that bystanders can play has been increasingly identified. This chapter explores different approaches to bystander training and the accumulating evidence for their effectiveness. It focuses particularly on the potential of arts-based approaches for engagement in bystander work, including an exploration of a theatre-based programme *You the Man* that is in use in the US and Australia, as well as examples from India and South Africa. Findings from ongoing research in the US and Australia illustrate the value of this type of approach in diverse settings including workplaces, sporting clubs, and educational institutions at both secondary and tertiary level.

Chapter 9 then considers the prevention of gender-based violence in faith communities. Effective programmes for the prevention of gender-based violence frequently involve community groups and organisations in order to maximise reach and impact. However, religious organisations have often been excluded from such efforts. While this may be explained by the fact that religious beliefs and practices have frequently been used to justify violence against women, the potential of religious organisations may be greater than is commonly perceived. As such, this chapter introduces a number of initiatives for the prevention of gender-based violence which have emerged in faith communities in different countries and explores the factors which facilitate the involvement of faith communities in these efforts.

Chapter 10 examines the potential contribution of health and social care professional practice to primary prevention. Moves towards person-centred practice with decision-making shared between patient/client and professional not only support the individual's autonomy in health matters, but also offer a powerful experience of respectful relationships and joint decision-making that can contribute to each of the three areas identified as important for preventing gender-based violence, namely promoting equal and respectful relationships between men and women; promoting non-violent social norms and reducing the effects of prior exposure to violence; and improving access to resources and systems of support. This chapter examines how the re-shaping of health and social care professional practice in relation to areas of practice as diverse as mental health, disability, management of chronic conditions and HIV/AIDS care shares common features with what is identified as helpful practice in relation to responding to domestic violence. These features include ensuring that the consultation provides a safe space, is empowering to the patient, that the patient is regarded as a full partner in the decision-making process, and respecting their autonomy. Such practice can be described as rights-based practice as well as person-centred.

Chapter 11 focuses on organisational gender equality work, exploring the rationale for asset-based approaches to preventing gender-based violence. It focuses particularly on work carried out using an asset-based approach in two organisations in rural Victoria, Australia. As a tool to guide the process involved in this work the steering committee chose the Interaction Gender Audit tool (Harvey and Morris 2010), one of the tools included in Gilles (2015). The process was intended to be as participatory as possible to build ownership of the resulting action plans for implementation in each organisation. The chapter explores the early stages of the work and the limited short-term evaluation of effectiveness.

References

Abramsky, T., Devries, K., Kiss, L., Nakuti, J., Kyegombe, N., Starmann, E., Cundill, B., Francisco, L., Kaye, D., Musuya, T., Michau, L. and Watts, C. (2014) 'Findings from the SASA! study: a cluster randomized controlled trial to assess the impact of a community mobilization intervention to prevent violence against women and reduce HIV risk in Kampala, Uganda', *BMC Medicine*, 12: 122. Doi: 10.1186/s12916-014-0122-5.

Abramsky, T., Devries, K.M., Michau, L., Nakuti, J., Musuya, T., Kiss, L., Kyegombe, N. and Watts, C. (2016a) 'Ecological pathways to prevention: how does the SASA! community mobilisation model work to prevent physical intimate partner violence against women?', *BMC Public Health*, 16: 339. Doi: 10.1186/s12889-016-3018-9.

Abramsky, T., Devries, K.M., Michau, L., Nakuti, J., Musuya, T., Kyegombe, N. and Watts, C. (2016b) 'The impact of SASA!, a community mobilisation intervention, on women's experiences of intimate partner violence: secondary findings from a cluster randomised trial in Kampala, Uganda', *Journal of Epidemiology and Community Health*, 270: 818–25.

Al-Shami, S.S.A., Razali, M.M., Majid, I., Rozelan, A. and Rashid, N. (2016) 'The effect of microfinance on women's empowerment: evidence from Malaysia', *Asian Journal of Women's Studies*, 22: 318–37.

Baird, S., McIntosh, C. and Özler, B. (2011) 'Cash or condition? Evidence from a cash transfer experiment', *Quarterly Journal of Economics*, 126: 1709–53.

Belsky, J. (1980) 'Child maltreatment: an ecological integration', *American Psychologist*, 35: 320–35.

Bronfenbrenner, U. (1979) *The Ecology of Human Development: experiments by nature and design*, Cambridge, MA: Harvard University Press.

Bronfenbrenner, U. (2005) *Making Human Beings Human: bioecological perspectives on human development*, Thousand Oaks, CA: Sage.

Carlson, B.E. (1984) 'Causes and maintenance of domestic violence: an ecological analysis', *Social Service Review*, 58: 569–87.

Carter, J. (2015) 'Patriarchy and violence against women and girls', *The Lancet*, 385: e40–1.

Cockburn, C. (2010) 'Gender relations as causal in militarization and war: a feminist standpoint', *International Feminist Journal of Politics*, 12: 139–57.

Cockburn, C. (2012) *Antimilitarism: political and gender dynamics of peace movements*, New York: Palgrave Macmillan.

Collins, P.H. (2015) 'Intersectionality's definitional dilemmas', *Annual Review of Sociology*, 41: 1–20.

Conway, P., Cox, P.J., Armstead, T.L., Ortega, S. and Cook-Craig, P.G. (2013) 'CDC's DELTA and EMPOWER programs: strengthening systems for primary prevention of intimate partner violence and sexual violence', in P. Conway, P.J. Cox, P.G. Cook-Craig, S. Ortega and T.L. Armstead (eds) *Strengthening Systems to Prevent Intimate Partner Violence and Sexual Violence*, London: Routledge.

Cooper-White, P. (1995) *The Cry of Tamar: violence against women and the church's response*, Minneapolis: Fortress Press.

Crenshaw, K. (1989) 'Demarginalizing the intersection of race and sex: a Black feminist critique of antidiscrimination doctrine, feminist theory and antiracist politics', *University of Chicago Legal Forum*, 140: 139–67.

Crenshaw, K. (1991) 'Mapping the margins: intersectionality, identity politics and violence against women of color', *Stanford Law Review*, 43: 1241–99.

Davis, R., Parks, L.F. and Cohen, L. (2006) *Sexual Violence and the Spectrum of Prevention: towards a community solution*, Enola, PA: National Sexual Violence Resource Centre.

Day, A., O'Leary, P., Chung, D. and Justo, D. (2009) *Domestic Violence: working with me. Research, practice experiences and integrated responses*, Annandale, NSW: The Federation Press.

Draucker, C. and Martsolf, D. (2010) 'Life-course typology of adults who experienced sexual violence', *Journal of Interpersonal Violence*, 25: 1155–82.

Duflo, E., Dupas, P., Kremer, M. and Sinei. S. (2006) *Education and HIV/AIDS Prevention: evidence from a randomized evaluation in western Kenya*. Policy Research Working Paper 4024, Washington, DC: World Bank.

Dutton, D.G. (1988) 'Profiling of wife assaulters: preliminary evidence for a tri-modal analysis', *Violence and Victims*, 5: 5–29.

Economic and Social Council (2013) *Commission on the Status of Women, report on the fifty-seventh session, 4–15 March 2013*, New York: United Nations. Online. Available at www.un.org/womenwatch/daw/csw/57sess.htm (accessed 1 December 2013).

Edleson, J. and Tolman, R.M. (1992) *Intervention for Men who Batter: an ecological approach*, Newbury Park, CA: Sage.

Ellsberg, M., Arango, D.J., Morton, M., Gennari, F., Kiplesund, S., Contreras, M. and Watts, C. (2015) 'Prevention of violence against women and girls: what does the evidence say?' *The Lancet*, 385: 1555–66.

Erulkar, A.S. and Muthengi, E. (2009) 'Evaluation of Berhane Hewan: a program to delay child marriage in rural Ethiopia', *International Perspectives on Sexual and Reproductive Health*, 35: 6–14.

Etherington, N.A. and Baker, L.L. (2016) *The Link between Boys' Victimization and Adult Perpetration of Intimate Partner Violence: opportunities for prevention across the life course*, London, Ontario: Centre for Research and Education on Violence against Women and Children.

Filemoni-Tofaeono, J.A. and Johnson, L. (2006) *Reweaving the Relational Mat: a Christian response to violence against women from Oceania*, London: Equionox.

Fleming, P.J., Gruskin, S., Rojo, F. and Dworkin, S.L. (2015) 'Men's violence against women and men are inter-related: recommendations for simultaneous intervention', *Social Science and Medicine*, 146: 249–56.

Fourth World Conference on Women (1995) *Beijing Declaration and Platform for Action*, United Nations. Online. Available at www.un.org/womenwatch/daw/beijing/platform/ (accessed 25 March 2016).

García-Moreno, C., Hegarty, K., Lucas d'Oliveira, A.F., Koziol-MacLain, J., Colombini, M. and Feder, G. (2015a) 'The health-systems response to violence against women', *The Lancet*, 385: 1567–79.

García-Moreno, C., Zimmerman, C., Morris-Gehring, A., Heise, L., Amin, A., Abrahams, N., Montoya, O., Bhate-Deosthali, P., Kilonzo, N. and Watts, C. (2015b) 'Addressing violence against women: a call to action', *The Lancet*, 385: 1685–95.

Gilles, K. (2015) *Pursuing Gender Equality Inside and Out: gender mainstreaming in international development organizations*, Washington, DC: Population Reference Bureau.

Gilligan, J. (2001) *Preventing Violence*, London: Thames and Hudson.

Guedes, A., Bott, S., Garcia-Moreno, C. and Colombini, M. (2016) 'Bridging the gaps: a global review of intersections of violence against women and violence against children', *Global Health Action*, 9: 31516. Doi: 10.3402/gha.v9.31516.

Hafner-Burton, E. and Pollack, M.A. (2002) 'Mainstreaming gender in global governance', *European Journal of International Relations*, 8: 339–73.

Hagemann-White, C., Kavemann, B., Kindler, H., Meysen, T., Puchert, R., Busche, M., Gabler, S., Grafe, B., Kungl, M., Schindler, G. and Schuck, H. (2010) *Review of Research on Factors at Play in Perpetration*. Online. Available at http://ec.europa.eu/justice/funding/daphne3/multi-level_interactive_model/understanding_perpetration_start_uinix.html (accessed 10 February 2017).

Hagemann-White, C., Kavemann, B., Kindler, H., Meysen, T., Puchert, R., Busche, M., Gabler, S., Grafe, B., Kungl, M., Schindler, G. and Schuck, H. (n.d.) *Factors conducive to violence against women, violence against children and sexual orientation violence and possible interventions.* Online. Available at http://ec.europa.eu/justice/funding/daphne3/multi-level_interactive_model/understanding_perpetration_start_uinix.html (accessed 10 February 2017).

Hansen, N. (2015) 'The development of psychological capacity for action: the empowering effect of a microfinance programme on women in Sri Lanka', *Journal of Social Issues*, 71: 597–613.

Harvey, J. and Morris, P. (2010) *The Gender Audit Handbook: a tool for organizational self-assessment and transformation*, Washington, DC: Interaction.

Haushofer, J. and Shapiro, J. (2013) *Household Response to Income Changes: evidence from an unconditional cash transfer program in Kenya*, New York: Give Directly. Online. Available at www.princeton.edu/~joha/publications/Haushofer_Shapiro_UCT_2013.pdf (accessed 18 February 2017).

Heise, L.L. (1998) 'Violence against women: an integrated ecological framework', *Violence against women*, 4: 262–90.

Hidrobo, M., Peterman, A. and Heise, L. (2015) *The Effect of Cash, Vouchers and Food Transfers on Intimate Partner Violence: evidence from a randomized experiment in Northern Ecuador*, Washington, DC: International Food Policy Research Institute.

Htun, M. and Weldon, S. (2012) 'The civic origins of progressive policy change: combatting violence against women in global perspective, 1975–2005', *American Political Science Review*, 106: 548–69.

InterAction-CAW and IIRR (2004) *Gender Mainstreaming in Action: successful innovations from Asia and the Pacific*, InterAction's Commission on the Advancement of Women and International Institute of Rural Reconstruction. Online. Available at www.interaction.org/document/gender-mainstreaming-action (accessed 17 February 2017).

James-Sebro, M. (2005) *Revealing the Power of Gender Mainstreaming: enhancing development effectiveness of non-governmental organizations in Africa*, Washington, DC: InterAction.

Jennings, W.G. and Reingle, J.M. (2012) 'On the number and shape of developmental/life-course violence, aggression, and delinquency trajectories: a state-of-the-art review', *Journal of Criminal Justice*, 40: 472–89.

Jewkes, R., Flood, M. and Lang, J. (2015) 'From work with men and boys to changes of social norms and reduction of inequities in gender relations: a conceptual shift in prevention of violence against women and girls', *The Lancet*, 385: 1580–9.

Kim, J.C., Watts, C.H., Hargreaves, J.R., Ndhlovu, L.X., Phetla, G., Morison, L.A., Busza, J., Porter, J.D.H. and Pronyk, P. (2007) 'Understanding the impact of a microfinance-based intervention on women's empowerment and the reduction of intimate partner violence in South Africa', *American Journal of Public Health*, 97: 1794–802.

Krug, E.G., Dahlberg, L.L., Mercy, J.A., Zwi, A.B. and Lozano, R. (eds) (2002) *World Report on Violence and Health*, Geneva: World Health Organization.

Kyegombe, N., Abramsky, T., Devries, K.M., Michau, L., Nakuti, J., Starmann, E., Musuya, T., Heise, L. and Watts, C. (2015) 'What is the potential for interventions designed to prevent violence against women to reduce children's exposure to violence? Findings from the SASA! Study, Kampala, Uganda', *Child Abuse and Neglect*, 50: 128–40.

Kyegombe, N., Starmann, E., Devries, K.M., Michau, L., Nakuti, J., Musuya, T., Watts, C. and Heise, L. (2014) 'SASA! is the medicine that treats violence: qualitative findings on how a community mobilisation intervention to prevent violence against women created change in Kampala, Uganda', *Global Health Action*, 7(1). Doi: 10.3402/gha.v7.25082.

Laing, L., Humphreys, C. and Cavanagh, K. (2013) *Social Work and Domestic Violence: developing critical and reflective practice*, London: Sage.

Lombardo, E. and Agustin, L.R. (2016) 'Intersectionality in European Union policymaking: the case of gender-based violence', *Politics*, 36: 364–73.

Macmillan, R. (2001) 'Violence and the life course: the consequences of victimization for personal and social development', *Annual Review of Sociology*, 27: 1–22.

Messina-Dysert, G. (2015) *Rape Culture and Spiritual Violence: religion, testimony and visions of healing*, London: Routledge.

Michau, L. (2008) *The SASA! Activist Kit for Preventing Violence against Women and HIV*, Kampala: Raising Voices. Online. Available at http://raisingvoices.org/sasa/ (accessed 15 February 2017).

Michau, L., Horn, J., Bank, A., Dutt, M. and Zimmerman, C. (2015) 'Prevention of violence against women and girls: lessons from practice', *The Lancet*, 385: 1672–84.

Moser, C. (2005) 'Has gender mainstreaming failed?', *International Feminist Journal of Politics*, 7: 576–90.

Murphy-Erby, Y., Christy-McMullin, K., Stauss, K. and Schriver, J. (2010) 'Multi-systems life course: a new practice perspective and its application in advanced practice with racial and ethnic populations,' *Journal of Human Behavior in the Social Environment*, 20: 672–87.

Nanda, P., Datta, N., Pradhan, E., Das, P. and Lamba, S. (2014) *Impact on Marriage: program assessment of conditional cash transfers*, Washington, DC: International Center for Research on Women.

Pollack, M.A. and Hafner-Burton, E. (2000) 'Mainstreaming gender in the European Union', *Journal of European Public Policy*, 7: 432–56.

Razavi, S. and Miller, C. (1995) *Gender Mainstreaming: a study of efforts by the UNDP, the World Bank and the ILO to institutionalize gender issues*. Occasional Paper 4, New York: United Nations Development Programme.

Rees, T. (2005) 'Reflections on the uneven development of gender mainstreaming in Europe', *International Feminist Journal of Politics*, 7: 555–74.

Shah, S., Tsitsou, L. and Woodin, S. (2016) 'Hidden voices: disabled women's experiences of violence and support over the life course', *Violence against Women*, 22(10): 1189–210.

Shahrokh, T. (2015) *Towards More Inclusive Strategies to Address Gender-Based Violence*, IDS Policy Briefing 104, Brighton, UK: Institute of Development Studies.

Stephens, A., Lewis, E.D. and Reddy, S. (2017) *Inclusive Systemic Evaluation for Gender Equality, Goals, Environments, and Voices from the Margins (ISE4GEMs): a guidance for evaluators for the SDG Era*, New York: UN Women.

Strid, S., Walby, S. and Armstrong, J. (2013) 'Intersectionality and multiple inequalities: visibility in British policy on violence against women', *Social Politics*, 20: 558–81.

True, J. and Mintrom, M. (2001) 'Transnational networks and policy diffusion: the case of gender mainstreaming', *International Studies Quarterly*, 45: 27–57.

United Nations (1993) *Declaration on the Elimination of Violence against Women*. Online. Available at www.un.org/documents/ga/res/48/a48r104.htm (accessed 10 February 2017).

UNDP (2007) *Gender Mainstreaming: a key driver of development in environment and energy. Training manual*, New York: United Nations Development Programme.

UN-HABITAT (2008) *Gender in Local Government: a sourcebook for trainers*, Nairobi, Kenya: United Nations Human Settlements Programme (UN-HABITAT).

UN Women (2014) *Guidance Note: gender mainstreaming in development programming*, New York: UN Women.

UN Women (n.d.) *About UN Women*. Online. Available at www.unwomen.org/en/about-us/about-un-women (accessed 5 March 2017).

Walby, S. (2005) 'Gender mainstreaming: productive tensions in theory and practice', *Social Politics*, 12: 321–43.

White, A.M. and Peretz, T. (2010) 'Emotions and redefining Black masculinity: movement narratives of two profeminist organizers', *Men and Masculinities*, 12: 403–24.

WHO (2011) *Gender Mainstreaming for Health Managers: a practical approach*, Geneva: World Health Organization.

2

WORKING WITH PARENTS AND YOUNG FAMILIES

Laura Coady, Ann Taket and Beth R. Crisp

Introduction

If a society-wide approach to preventing gender-based violence is to have any lasting effect, it must reach into the relationships most intricately woven into our lives, the most intimate of shared spaces. A young family is one such space: becoming parents transforms a couple's relationship, bringing sudden changes, intense emotions and physical intimacy. As such it is alive with the risk of violence which can reverberate through generations but there is also the potential for intergenerational change.

This chapter will examine some recent initiatives that work with young families to prevent gender-based violence, beginning with programmes – both universal and those targeted at 'at-risk' groups – for new and expectant parents. We will look at parenting programmes that work with people considered especially at risk of gender-based violence. Finally, we will take an in-depth look at an Australian relationship education programme, *Baby Makes 3*.

Families should not be considered in isolation from their community and broader society. While parenthood has some universal qualities, there are distinct pressures, expectations and stressors that bear down on particular individuals, families and locations, different strengths and investments, and different meanings attached to family and parenthood. Nevertheless, several overviews (for example Ellsberg et al. 2015; Fulu et al. 2014; Webster and Flood 2015) have deemed the general approach of working with new parents to be promising in preventing gender-based violence, whether directly (as measured by levels of violence before and after an intervention) or – more commonly – in their success in removing or minimising risk factors, or establishing and strengthening protective factors.

However, there are limitations to any generalisations, owing to the diversity of programmes and outcomes, a lack of longitudinal studies in such a new field, and the often limited resources of evaluators (Wessels et al. 2013). Most evaluated programmes are from high-income countries (Ellsberg et al. 2015), and many initiatives – if only by default – work predominantly with married, middle-class, white, heterosexual couples (Dion 2005; Hawkins et al. 2008a).

Meta-analyses and large-scale reviews have, however, identified elements common to many successful violence-prevention programmes, including the need to address underlying risk factors related to gender inequality (Fulu et al. 2014; Our Watch 2015; Webster and Flood 2015); the need for a clear theory of change to drive programme design (Fulu et al. 2014; Wessels et al. 2013); the value of multiple components (Ellsberg et al. 2015; Fulu et al. 2014); the involvement of multiple sectors and stakeholders (Ellsberg et al. 2015; Our Watch 2015; Webster and Flood 2015); the inclusion of skill-building exercises (Fulu et al. 2014); the use of trained professionals to facilitate the programme (Wessels et al. 2013); and the involvement of both parents in the programme (Fulu et al. 2014).

Not all promising initiatives are motivated by a desire to prevent gender-based violence. For instance, some couples' relationship workshops are primarily designed to keep marriages intact (if appropriate) during the stressful transition to parenthood. Gender-based violence may not be directly addressed (and 'conflict' couched in gender-neutral and non-violent terms), but the programmes can still show promising results in reducing couple dissatisfaction, and in strengthening communication and conflict-resolution skills, all of which are known to reduce the likelihood of violence.

Working with expectant and new parents

Bringing a child into the world can be an intense experience for parents, steeped in hope, joy, pain, love, stress, uncertainty and fatigue, and marked by rapid changes. The period leading up to the birth and up to 12 months after has been identified as a stage of life that increases conflict within intimate relationships (Glade et al. 2005) and, relatedly, as a period with a high prevalence of intimate partner violence (IPV) (Halford et al. 2011). The key changes for couples consistently noted by researchers are: cohabiting heterosexual couples switching to more traditional gender roles, especially in their division of household labour and childcare; an increase in conflict within the relationship; and reduced feelings of relationship satisfaction (Glade et al. 2005). Postnatal depression, anxiety, low self-esteem and social isolation are also common, affecting women more commonly and severely than men. Each factor alone has been linked to an increased likelihood of gender-based violence (Heise 2011). Compounding such factors leaves young families vulnerable to the emergence of violence even before other external stressors are considered.

However, the perinatal stage also opens up opportunities for prevention efforts. People who are otherwise hard to reach generally make contact with health services, exposing them to support and programmes they might not otherwise have sought (Hunter and Commerford 2015; Petch et al. 2012). Most parents want what is best for their children, which may explain why – beyond medical necessity – they are more open at this time to interventions that explore such sensitive subjects as good parenting and healthy intimate relationships (Moore and Florsheim 2008).

Preventative programmes involving young families can short-circuit cycles of violence in a number of potent ways. Preventing a child from witnessing gender-based violence in the home is not only a good in itself, but might also help to interrupt their own potential trajectory towards violence (Heise 2011; Our Watch 2015).

Couples' relationship education

The most common form of preventative intervention during the transition to parenthood is couples' relationship education (CRE). Usually consisting of facilitated group workshops, this focuses on improving couples' communication and conflict-resolution knowledge and skills, so building up the protective factors that can buffer, and even directly minimise, the risk factors present in the transition to parenthood. A meta-analysis by Pinquart and Teubert (2010) found small but positive effects of CRE on communication, psychological wellbeing and couple adjustment. Stronger effects were likely if programmes ran for five or more sessions, involved both antenatal and postnatal components, were run by professionals, and worked to develop realistic shared expectations of parenthood, enhanced couple communication and mutual support.

Hunter and Commerford (2015) summarise various meta-analyses with the conclusion that CRE generally produces good results for couples, but caution that most evaluations do not measure long-term effects and cannot be considered universally applicable, especially because most programmes work overwhelmingly with married couples who considered themselves happy in their relationships. Since higher levels of relationship distress and external stressors are understood to worsen the outcome of such generalised programmes, there is clearly an opportunity for CRE specific to the often distressing time of new parenthood.

Most CRE programmes addressing known risk factors for gender-based violence in new families do so without explicitly aiming to prevent or reduce violence (see for example Charles et al. 2014; Clark et al. 2013; Wood et al. 2014). One example is *Bringing Baby Home* (Shapiro and Gottman 2005; Shapiro et al. 2015), a short two-day psycho-communicative-educational intervention aimed at helping expectant and new parents to 'make a smooth, positive transition to becoming a family' (Shapiro and Gottman 2005: 7). The intervention involved lectures, role-play and skill-building exercises around what to expect in the relationship through the transition, as well as conflict-handling skills, maintenance of friendship and intimacy, and practical information about childhood development. An evaluation revealed significant positive results over time compared with a control group in all the intended outcome areas: marital quality, postpartum depression and observed marital hostility. Analysis also revealed that changes can be gradual and complex in their unfolding, and that it may be easier to build up the positive elements of relationships than to remove the negative. This latter point reaffirms the need for primary prevention to occur as early as possible, and underlines the efficacy of strengths-based intervention models; see for example Scerra (2011) and Herrenkohl et al. (2015).

Schulz et al. (2006) detail a much more extensive programme to prevent couple dysfunction across the transition to parenthood, *Becoming a Parent*. For 24 weeks across antenatal and postnatal periods, groups of couples engaged in semi-structured discussions led by pairs of married clinical psychologists. Topics included how participants saw their relationship, division of family labour, communication styles, ideas about parenting and actual parenting styles, work and social support outside the family, and the influence of their own experiences growing up. The programme provided a safe space for couples to confront, share and explore the challenges that come with parenthood and develop and test their own solutions. Compared with a control group, it significantly slowed normal marital decline over five years.

Hawkins et al. (2008b) describe *Marriage Moments*, which – distinct from most programmes – is mostly self-guided, completed by couples together at their own pace using a video and manual covering the foundations of healthy relationships, and concepts of fairness and justice in relationships. An evaluation of the impact of attaching this CRE component to a parenting-focused curriculum found that *Marriage Moments* did not in fact increase relationship satisfaction, but did as an offshoot increase the father's involvement in daily childcare. This was understood to indicate that at least some core messages about healthy relationship foundations were being absorbed and acted upon, albeit in unanticipated ways.

In spite of the wealth of CRE programmes on offer to new parents, only a small number are designed explicitly to prevent gender-based violence. One example is *Becoming Parents* (Tiwari et al. 2011), a partnership between hospitals, social workers and community volunteers in Hong Kong. Its working notion was that easing the stress of transition to parenthood would lessen the risk of gender-based violence. Three antenatal sessions offered information, discussion and skill-building exercises around engaged fatherhood, communication and shared infant care, and adjusting to parenthood. After the birth, trained volunteers offered new parents weekly peer support for three months. The programme reduced depressive symptoms in fathers (though not mothers) and improved parental competence via standardised measurements, with very positive self-reporting by participants of the programme's impact on marital satisfaction, communication skills and parental competence (Tiwari et al. 2011, n.d).

Targeted prevention initiatives

Another approach to preventing gender-based violence within young families is to target those who are especially 'at risk' of violence due to amplifying stressors or circumstances (for an overview of risk factors see Heise 2011; Our Watch 2015). Risk factors most commonly addressed in the literature are being unmarried

(Wood et al. 2014), young (Florsheim et al. 2011; Wise and David 2014), economically disadvantaged (Bradley et al. 2011; Charles et al. 2014), and having already experienced intimate partner violence (Bradford et al. 2011; Bradley et al. 2011; Wilde and Doherty 2011). Many programmes create an umbrella term such as 'high-risk' or 'vulnerable', acknowledging the diversity of risks and their possible overlaps.

Teenage mothers are under-represented in prevention services despite being particularly vulnerable to stress and intimate partner violence during and after pregnancy (Silverman et al. 2006). The *Young Parenthood Program* (*YPP*), a co-parent counselling programme for pregnant teenagers and their young (under 24) male co-parents providing an average of 10 antenatal sessions with a trained counsellor, allowed young parents to identify their needs and strengths as co-parents, and to develop the interpersonal skills needed to create a supportive and non-violent co-parenting relationship. Compared with a more universal programme, *YPP* was able to address issues especially pertinent to young parents, such as unplanned pregnancy and difficulty verbalising emotions (Florsheim et al. 2011). This programme is rare not only in seeking explicitly to prevent violence by participants, but also in measuring its occurrence and severity across three time points. It yielded promising results, with young parents randomly assigned to the programme significantly less likely to experience or perpetrate IPV than the control group, though the strength of the finding diminished over time.

As with universal programmes, targeted interventions can be ineffective or have negative outcomes if they do not adequately anticipate and address the diversity of potential participants and the complex histories they live with. For example, Wood et al. (2012, 2014) explore how *Building Strong Families*, adapted from promising universal CRE programmes to target low-income, unmarried, expectant or new parents, failed to meet any of its expected outcomes and in fact generated some negative results. Recognising that group members may have had negative educational experiences, the facilitators avoided didactic presentations and instead facilitated collaborative discussions and offered support in areas such as employment, mental health and education. Yet it failed to improve the quality of couple relationships or co-parenting, or enhance father involvement. In some cases it fared worse than the control group: couples were less likely to stay together, and fathers less likely to spend regular time with their children or provide financial support.

Wood et al. theorise that there may not have been enough sensitivity or nuance in the messages about what constitutes a 'good relationship' and a 'good parent' for this particular group. One key message taken by *Building Strong Families* participants was that fathers needed to 'step up'. Facing significant stresses and structural disadvantages, some men may have felt they could not meet those expectations, leading to a sense of failure and a feeling that it would be best to 'withdraw from these relationships' (Wood et al. 2014: 461). At one Baltimore site with particularly negative outcomes, fathers blamed themselves and their problems for the relationship breakdown more than did the control group, despite no difference in actual socio-economic circumstances.

In light of this, Wood et al. (2014) suggested running an employment programme alongside the relationship education, and offering a more realistic version of parenthood, fathering and relationships to aspire to. One programme that adopted this expanded approach, *Strong Couples–Strong Children*, produced significant positive results (Charles et al. 2014). By combining relationship education, coordinated access to family, employment and education services and fatherhood support services with male mentors, the programme aimed to help remove external environmental stressors in participants' lives, not least to provide the time and space necessary to work on strengthening family relationships.

Difficulties and dangers remain in establishing who is 'at risk' – and in assuming who is not – in any general population of new parents. One of the most promising avenues takes a stepped-care approach (Halford and Petch 2010), starting as a universal programme open to all new parents, offering a basic assessment of relationships and generalised healthy relationship education, then offering more intensive training, education and home visits to those who desire it or are assessed to be at higher risk of relationship distress or violence for any reason. This is deemed to be cost efficient, and avoids presuming any neatly defined 'at-risk' attributions from the start.

Parenting programmes

While focusing on healthy relationships can reduce at-risk parenting, many violence-prevention initiatives for young families are designed with child protection foremost in mind, and focus on improving parenting capacities and skills rather than the parental relationship. Approaches include education programmes, home visitation and support, and screening and treatment of parents for risk factors around child abuse and maltreatment.

Parenting programmes can significantly reduce child maltreatment and abuse (Chen and Chan 2016). Wessels et al. (2013) summarised the common qualities of successful programmes, which include: sound programme theory; delivery when participants are most receptive to change, such as early childhood; opportunities to practise new skills; teaching positive parenting strategies; and considering the difficulties between adults in the family.

Haggerty et al. (2013: 239) found that parenting programmes that successfully addressed child behaviour intervened early, and provided 'opportunities for meaningful involvement; skills; rewards, recognition, reinforcement; bonding; and clear expectations for behaviour'. One example, *Positive Parenting Program*, was developed in Australia and run in a variety of countries. A flexible system with a stepped-care approach, its intent is to 'promote positive parenting and to reduce the risk of child abuse and neglect through promoting safe and engaging environments, creating positive learning environments, using effective discipline, creating clear and reasonable expectations, and self-care for parents' (Haggerty et al. 2013: 233).

Baby Makes 3: a case study

In the second half of this chapter we explore one particular programme, *Baby Makes 3 (BM3)*, an education programme for new parents designed explicitly to help prevent violence against women. As a primary prevention initiative aimed universally at all new first-time parents, it is an especially interesting case study as, rather than just working on elements in intimate relationships that are associated with gender-based violence, such as increased stress and relationship dissatisfaction, *BM3* aims to directly address the key driver of violence against women across cultures and communities, namely gender inequity. *Baby Makes 3* was originally developed by Whitehorse Community Health Service (now Carrington Health) and the City of Whitehorse, in the eastern suburbs of Melbourne, with funding from VicHealth (Flynn 2011).

The Victorian Department of Justice and Regulation under its initiative to support primary prevention and early intervention-focused partnership projects then funded an expanded programme, *Baby Makes 3 Plus*, in the Great South Coast rural region of Victoria. In addition to the provision of the *BM3* programme to new parents across the region, skills training in gender equity and in the identification of women at risk of gender-based violence was provided for health professionals and organisations involved in early-years care. While this 'Plus' component represents a good example of multi-component programming, with trainees and stakeholders finding it helped build greater capacity to deliver *BM3* and to support other preventative initiatives in the region, the focus here will be on the core relationship education programme as it was delivered in the Great South Coast region.

Baby Makes 3 relationship education programme

BM3 was offered as part of local council-run maternal and child health services across the region. All first-time parents were invited and encouraged by child and maternal health nurses to attend what was described to them as a 'healthy relationships' programme with their partner and child. Delivered by two facilitators – specifically one male and one female – the free programme consisted of three two-hour evening sessions held over consecutive weeks. Facilitators guided structured group discussions and activities around the following key topics: the lifestyle and relationship changes following the birth of a child; gendered expectations of new mums and new dads; gendered division of household labour and childcare; equality as the basis of a healthy relationship; building intimacy after the birth of a child; dealing with conflict; and communication skills. Discussion took place with the group as a whole or in breakout mothers and fathers groups. Sessions were supplemented and reinforced by a number of take-home exercises for couples to complete together between and beyond the three sessions.

Theory of change and expected impacts

The design of *BM3* was underpinned by a theory of change (see Flynn 2011: 19) that mapped out how the programme would meet its direct objective of increasing participating parents' capacity to build equal and respectful relationships in response to the lifestyle and relationship changes that follow the birth of a child, and thus how it would meet the broader objective of primary prevention of gender-based violence by way of increasing gender equity (Taket et al. 2016).

Specific short-, medium- and long-term impacts were anticipated and expected to build on from one another. Launching from awareness and understanding about gender equality gained by couples' participation in the programme activities, short-term impacts were expected to be that men and women would develop a shared language to describe and discuss changes they were experiencing through the transition to parenthood, indicated by improved communication, and that participants would experience a shift in attitudes marked by increased understanding of their partner's experience and greater support for gender equality. Medium-term impacts were anticipated to be behavioural changes in how couples structured their parenting roles and relationships. Finally, the long-term impact was theorised to be that couples would restructure their roles and relationships in demonstration of greater understanding, respect and equality.

This theory of change is supported by a number of researchers in the field (for example Fulu et al. 2014; Webster and Flood 2015). It is argued that relationship education initiatives need to incorporate gender analyses into their programme design, and should aim to be gender-transformative, if they are to help in preventing gender-based violence. If programmes involving relationships between men and women are approached in gender-neutral terms, they may 'inadvertently compound gender inequality and hence be harmful to women' (Webster and Flood 2015: 68) because the gendered power dynamics in relationships, and the broader social climate of gender inequality that drives and excuses violence against women, remain unacknowledged and thus unaddressed.

This seems especially pertinent in regard to relationship education programmes around the transition to parenthood. While many programmes identify the heightened stress levels, hostility, conflict, social isolation and relationship dissatisfaction that routinely come with the birth of a child as issues for couples to resolve, far fewer interrogate or attempt to remedy the imbalanced gender expectations and intense social pressures that likely give rise to many of these risk factors for violence. This is in spite of plentiful evidence (see Glade et al. 2005 for an overview) that much stress and conflict during this time for heterosexual couples revolves around the division of household labour and the adoption of traditional, fixed parenting roles, two areas steeped in highly gendered expectations and long-entrenched inequality between genders.

Evaluation of impacts

As well as researching and assessing economic impact, standardised health out-comes, and the reach, adoption, implementation and maintenance of the *BM3* as it was delivered in the Great South Coast, external evaluators sought evidence about actual changes in awareness, attitudes, skills and behaviours among the participants of the programme (Taket et al. 2016), in order to examine whether there were posi-tive impacts in line with the programme's theory of change.

Drawing on multiple sources of data in the form of in-depth interviews with participants, facilitators and other stakeholders, group evaluation forms and ques-tionnaires to parents pre- and post-programme, the evaluation identified promising positive impacts, along with a few challenges and tensions to consider and poten-tially resolve for any future implementation of the programme.

What worked

> I was really impressed with it, probably because I hadn't really been in a group situation like that before. I definitely enjoyed the parts where the men were separated from the women and then they were brought back into the room to discuss the same answers, and that was really insightful . . . I've kept in touch with a couple of blokes from the course . . . [People] shared some brilliant stories and some great experiences and that time to actually tell their story I think was really cathartic for a lot of people, and added to that grow-ing sense of confidence, that things are going to be all right and that we're doing the right thing.
>
> *(Father, interview)*

> It is great. Makes you think of things that you may not have thought about before. Opens discussion.
>
> *(Mother, group programme evaluation form)*

These two quotes illustrate the high level of satisfaction reported by almost all parents on the programme, with positive impacts reported up to 15 months after completion (interviews were carried out between 3 and 15 months after pro-gramme completion). These impacts included changes in awareness, attitudes, skills and behaviour that directly support gender equity, and corresponded to each of the different stages and indicators of change in the theory of change model underlying the *BM3* programme design.

Important changes included increased awareness of societal expectations of mothers and the extent of caring and domestic responsibilities assumed by them. These in turn produced changes in behaviour, such as mothers adjusting their expectations of themselves, and fathers prioritising family over work and contribut-ing more towards household tasks and childcare. All of these positive changes can be seen as supporting increased gender equity.

Parents, both mothers and fathers, relished the opportunity to talk with and listen to other parents in a safe space. The programme provided the chance to open up difficult but important conversations between partners. Other important impacts were experienced within the couple relationship, with parents reporting enhanced communication and conflict-resolution skills, and an increased focus on the relationship. One mother illustrated this as she talked about how what she learnt in the programme had helped her and her partner through a particularly difficult period that occurred six months after the end of the programme:

> It was a very stressful fortnight and that was probably the most alien we'd felt to each other ever and for the first time ever, I didn't really feel like I could talk to him about it and I just thought, well I've just got to look after this baby, whatever I'll just see you on the other side of this. And that was unusual for me. But then . . . I do remember thinking at some point about the things that we'd learnt at *Baby Makes 3*. It was like the, 'You did this to me' kind of language. So the language he [facilitator] taught us to say, 'I feel'. I certainly used that in that week and said, 'I feel like we're not getting along very well this week and we need to because we won't make it otherwise.' And by not make it, I mean we'll have a blow up. So, yeah, our relationship did change for a few weeks but we certainly had the right tools this time to get through it and come back and now I think we're pretty much back where we were.

A further impact was the social connections parents made and maintained as a result of participating in *Baby Makes 3*; this connected to the value of the programme in normalising the challenges they were facing as new parents. Improved social connectedness is important for protection and promotion of health, and is particularly key for those living in rural and regional contexts.

The evaluation identified the importance of a mixed gender facilitation team for successful programme delivery. The evaluation findings also identified the importance to parents of diversity in the programme group, as they appreciated the opportunity to hear different viewpoints and responses to the common challenges they experience as new parents. This implies that is is important to provide the programme to all new parents, rather than as a programme targeted at those at high risk. Exceptions to this were suggested as being necessary for two particular groups, Indigenous parents and young parents, who were under-represented in the Great South Coast programme attendances. It was argued that these specific groups within the larger group of new parents would benefit from specialised and particular programmes to reflect highly particular circumstances not captured by a universalist programme, for example, because of Indigenous parents having broader conceptions of family, along with compounded risk of family violence and complicated intergenerational trauma from colonial violence and racism, and younger parents not relating to the family life of more settled, economically stable older parents, and perhaps potentially being more receptive to shorter, more informal programmes. Tension between universal and targeted options will probably always exist in public health initiatives, and this is not necessarily a bad thing: it keeps questions alive about what constitutes good public health, and for whom, and who is included in our conception of 'the universal'.

The challenge of boosting uptake

Across the two full years for which data was available (2014–15) between 18 and 29 per cent of all new parents in the five local government areas attended the programme, the overall average being 21 per cent. This level of uptake can be considered as reasonable given factors such as shift work, farm work and fly-in–fly-out work that are important features of much of the employment in the region, coupled with long travel distances necessary to reach the programme delivery venues.

Analysis of uptake rates for *Baby Makes 3* over its first year led to the suggestion of a brief introductory session in the antenatal setting, so that fathers-to-be could be introduced directly to the idea of the programme. A pilot of this arrangement was carried out in the town of Portland from January 2015 and was very successful. The reaction of fathers to the session was extremely positive; all of the fathers interviewed went on to attend the postnatal programme with their partners and all reported that the decision to attend the postnatal session was made mutually with their partners and influenced by the antenatal session. The positive effect of the antenatal session echoes findings in the literature from research into other parent education programmes (for example Coster et al. 2015; Florsheim et al. 2011; Tiwari et al. 2011, n.d.). Antenatal sessions were also suggested as a valuable addition by parents who had not experienced them, by programme facilitators, and by maternal and child health staff. The facilitators and maternal and child health staff linked this suggestion explicitly to improving uptake.

Other suggestions for tackling low uptake included finding different ways of directly inviting fathers to the programme, more widespread publicity about it and investigating an alternative, concentrated form of delivery in one or two daytime sessions held at weekends.

The challenge of perceived negativity towards men

One possible negative effect of the programme lay in it being regarded as directed against men or negative about men. This was an issue that was raised unprompted by a small number of parents in the interviews, the analysis of facilitators' forms and a small number of the group programme evaluation forms completed by parents. In the interviews with facilitators and stakeholders conducted from July to September 2015, the issue was specifically explored if the participant had not raised it in response to open questions.

This issue was raised unprompted by four of the 10 facilitators interviewed, and all but one facilitator interviewed had noticed some of their group participants perceive elements of negativity towards men. In at least one case this had resulted in the couple choosing not to attend the third session of the programme, with the female partner reporting in her interview:

> I know a lot of the males felt it was very critical towards the fathers. Yeah, so that's why we didn't go back for the last session, my partner just didn't – he didn't want to deal with it anymore like, it was very critical towards the dads, there was no sort of positive things, like, they didn't refer to anything positive regarding the fathers.

Other parents who discussed this reported some discomfort. This points to the need for maintaining a style of programme delivery that challenges those present to think about gender equity without compromising their participation, or the benefits achieved from it. Many facilitators felt that more training and skills were needed to deliver the programme more confidently and effectively, that training needed to be refreshed beyond the initial session and that ongoing discussion about the facilitation process and experience would be useful. It seems especially vital to ensure that facilitators feel adequately prepared for dealing with discomfort and defensiveness, and have an outlet to debrief about any challenges, especially around the issue of perceived negativity towards men. While the current manual discusses the issue of resistance from fathers, it would be helpful to expand the coverage of possible strategies to respond to this within the manual.

Single parents, unaccompanied parents

Challenges to successful implementation are also posed by the presence of single parents and lone parents (those whose partner is absent). In analysis of the group programme evaluation forms, a small number of single mothers reported that the programme was less relevant to them (although some reported it was useful). One single mother reported that she had sometimes felt awkward; this was echoed by a number of facilitators who sensed discomfort and awkwardness from some single mothers in their sessions. During the course of the project, facilitators developed ways of modifying delivery and activities to accommodate single and lone parents, and it would be beneficial to incorporate this into a revision of the programme manual.

Conclusions

The overall cost to the service provider was A$582 per couple in the rural region of the Great South Coast (compared with A$325 per couple in metropolitan Melbourne), a relatively low figure in view of the range of positive impacts produced. A particularly important feature in programme delivery was using a pair of facilitators (male and female). Minimal possible negative effects were identified, and the experience gained in programme delivery should enable these to be further reduced in the future.

The evaluation identified the importance of good working relationships between programme providers and maternal and child health staff, as well as the importance of wider partnerships with other stakeholders. Other stakeholders reported very positive views about the programme, for example a community service agency staff member said:

> I think the *Baby Makes 3* is quite an outstanding model . . . it's sort of best practice primary prevention because you don't even need to have the conversation per se about violence. Your focus is more on equality and respect.

A maternal and child health nurse explained how she saw it:

> having a man there and being there for the dads, I think that really works well, because the dads can tend to get forgotten. When you have a baby, it's all focused on the mum . . . and the dads are on the sidelines . . . [S]ome of the feedback I've had is that the dads get a lot out of it, especially meeting other dads . . . Dads are meeting dads and they can talk about how it is for them.

There were considerable advantages to organising delivery of the *Baby Makes 3* programme on a region-wide basis, rather than separate programmes in each of the five local government areas, some of which reported very few births per annum. *BM3* showed that it is possible to successfully run a transition-to-parenthood relationship programme that has gender equity as an explicit discussion point and broad goal. Positive impacts, including increase in gender equity within participating couples, are promising, and will hopefully be more rigorously tested and replicated in future research. As such these conclusions are very consistent with those reached in the original (metropolitan) evaluation of *Baby Makes 3* (Flynn 2011), and demonstrate the programme's applicability in a rural and regional setting. While most of the challenges identified above can easily be addressed in future programme delivery, the programme remains firmly oriented around parenting in heterosexual couples. Same-sex couples are not included in the heteronormative language of the programme and gendered analyses of couple dynamics.

References

Bradford, K.P., Skogrand, L. and Higginbotham, B.J. (2011) 'Intimate partner violence in a statewide couple and relationship education initiative', *Journal of Couple and Relationship Therapy*, 10: 169–84.

Bradley, R.P.C., Friend, D.J. and Gottman, J.M. (2011) 'Supporting healthy relationships in low-income, violent couples: reducing conflict and strengthening relationship skills and satisfaction', *Journal of Couple and Relationship Therapy*, 10: 97–116.

Charles, P., Jones, A. and Guo, S. (2014) 'Treatment effects of a relationship-strengthening intervention for economically disadvantaged new parents', *Research on Social Work Practice*, 24: 321–38.

Chen, M. and Chan, K.L. (2016) 'Effects of parenting programs on child maltreatment prevention: a meta-analysis', *Trauma, Violence, and Abuse*, 17: 88–104.

Clark, C., Young, M.S. and Dow, M.G. (2013) 'Can strengthening parenting couples' relationships reduce at-risk parenting attitudes?', *The Family Journal*, 21: 306–12.

Coster, D., Brookes, H. and Sanger, C. (2015) *Evaluation of the Baby Steps Programme: pre- and post-measures study*, London: NSPCC.

Dion, M.R. (2005) 'Healthy marriage programs: learning what works', *The Future of Children*, 15: 139–56.

Ellsberg, M., Aranjo, D.J., Morton, M., Gennari, F., Kiplesund, S., Contreras, M. and Watts, C. (2015) 'Prevention of violence against women and girls: what does the evidence say?', *The Lancet*, 385: 1555–66.

Florsheim, P., McArthur, L., Hudak, C., Heavin, S. and Burrow-Sanchez, J. (2011) 'The Young Parenthood Program: preventing intimate partner violence between adolescent mothers and young fathers', *Journal of Couple and Relationship Therapy*, 10: 117–34.

Flynn, D. (2011) *Baby Makes 3: project report*, Box Hill, Victoria: Whitehorse Community Health Service.

Fulu, E., Kerr-Wilson, A. and Lang, J. (2014) *What Works to Prevent Violence against Women and Girls? Evidence review of interventions to prevent violence against women and girls (Annex F)*. Online. Available at www.gov.uk/government/publications/what-works-in-preventing-violence-against-women-and-girls-review-of-the-evidence-from-the-programme (accessed 25 November 2016).

Glade, A.C., Bean, R.A. and Vira, R. (2005) 'A prime time for marital/relational intervention: a review of the transition to parenthood literature with treatment recommendations', *American Journal of Family Therapy*, 33: 319–36.

Haggerty, K.P., McGlynn-Wright, A. and Klima, T. (2013) 'Promising parenting programmes for reducing adolescent problem behaviours', *Journal of Children's Services*, 8: 229–43.

Halford, W.K. and Petch, J. (2010) 'Couple psychoeducation for new parents: observed and potential effects on parenting', *Clinical Child and Family Psychology Review*, 13: 164–80.

Halford, W.K., Petch, J., Creedy, D.K. and Gamble, J. (2011) 'Intimate partner violence in couples seeking relationship education for the transition to parenthood', *Journal of Couple and Relationship Therapy*, 10: 152–68.

Hawkins, A.J., Blanchard, V.L., Baldwin, S.A. and Fawcett, E.B. (2008a) 'Does marriage and relationship education work? A meta-analytic study', *Journal of Consulting and Clinical Psychology*, 76: 723–34.

Hawkins, A.J., Lovejoy, K.R., Holmes, E.K., Blanchard, V.L. and Fawcett, E. (2008b) 'Increasing fathers' involvement in child care with a couple-focused intervention during the transition to parenthood', *Family Relations*, 57: 49–59.

Heise, L.L. (2011) *What Works to Prevent Partner Violence? An evidence overview*, London: STRI VE. Online. Available at http://strive.lshtm.ac.uk/system/files/attachments/What%20works%20to%20prevent%20partner%20violence.pdf (accessed 24 November 2016).

Herrenkohl, T.I., Higgins, D.J., Merrick, M.T. and Leeb, R.T. (2015) 'Positioning a public health framework at the intersection of child maltreatment and intimate partner violence: primary prevention requires working outside existing systems', *Child Abuse and Neglect*, 48: 22–8.

Hunter, C. and Commerford, J. (2015) *Relationship Education and Counselling: recent research findings*. CFCA paper 33, Melbourne: Australian Institute of Family Studies.

Moore, D.R. and Florsheim, P. (2008) 'Interpartner conflict and child abuse risk among African American and Latino adolescent parenting couples', *Child Abuse and Neglect*, 32: 463–75.

Our Watch (2015) *Change the Story: a shared framework for the primary prevention of violence against women and their children in Australia*, Melbourne: Our Watch, ANROWS and Victorian Health Promotion Foundation.

Petch, J., Halford, W.K., Creedy, D.K. and Gamble, J. (2012) 'Couple relationship education at the transition to parenthood: a window of opportunity to reach high-risk couples', *Family Process*, 51: 498–511.

Pinquart, M. and Teubert, D. (2010) 'A meta-analytic study of couple interventions during the transition to parenthood', *Family Relations*, 59: 221–31.

Scerra, N. (2011) *Strengths-based Practice: the evidence*, Parramatta, NSW: UnitingCare Children, Young People and Families.

Schulz, M.S., Cowan, C.P. and Cowan, P.A. (2006) 'Promoting healthy beginnings: a randomized controlled trial of a preventive intervention to preserve marital quality during the transition to parenthood', *Journal of Consulting and Clinical Psychology*, 74: 20–31.

Shapiro, A.F. and Gottman, J.M. (2005) 'Effects on marriage of a psycho-communicative-educational intervention with couples undergoing the transition to parenthood, evaluation at 1-year post intervention', *Journal of Family Communication*, 5: 1–24.

Shapiro, A.F., Gottman, J.M. and Fink, B.C. (2015) 'Short-term change in couples' conflict following a transition to parenthood intervention', *Couple and Family Psychology: Research and Practice*, 4: 239–51.

Silverman, J.G., Decker, M.R., Reed, E. and Raj, A. (2006) 'Intimate partner violence victimization prior to and during pregnancy among women residing in 26 US states: associations with maternal and neonatal health', *American Journal of Obstetrics and Gynecology*, 195: 140–8.

Taket, A., Busst, C., Coady, L. and Crisp, B. (2016) *The Baby Makes 3 Project in the Great South Coast Region: final report from the external evaluation January 2016*, Melbourne: Deakin University.

Tiwari, A., Wong, J.Y.H. and Yuen, F.K.H. (2011) *Positive Fathering: a programme to enhance the mental health and marital relationship of expectant couples*, Hong Kong: University of Hong Kong.

Tiwari, A., Leung, W.C., Chow, K.M., Yuk, H., Fong, D.Y.T., Yuen, F.K.H. and Tolman, R. (n.d.) *Becoming Parents: a hospital–community partnership to enhance transition to parenthood*, Hong Kong: University of Hong Kong.

Webster, K. and Flood, M. (2015) *Framework Foundations 1: a review of the evidence on correlates of violence against women and what works to prevent it*, Melbourne: OurWatch, VicHealth, ANROWS.

Wessels, I., Mikton, C., Ward, C.L., Kilbane, T., Alves, R., Campello, G., Dubowitz, H., Hutchings, J., Jones, L., Lynch, M. and Madrid, B. (2013) *Preventing Violence: evaluating outcomes of parenting programmes*, Geneva: World Health Organization.

Wilde, J.L. and Doherty, W.J. (2011) 'Intimate partner violence between unmarried parents before and during participation in a couple and relationship education program', *Journal of Couple and Relationship Therapy*, 10: 135–51.

Wise, S. and David, L. (2014) *An Outcomes and Process Evaluation of the 'Hey Babe' Early Parenting Support Program*, Melbourne: Anglicare Victoria.

Wood, R.G., Moore, Q., Clarkwest, A., Killewald, A. and Monahan, S. (2012) *The Long-Term Effects of Building Strong Families: a relationship skills education program for unmarried parents. OPRE Report # 2012-28A*, Washington, DC: Office of Planning, Research and Evaluation, Administration for Children and Families, US Department of Health and Human Services.

Wood, R.G., Moore, Q., Clarkwest, A. and Killewald, A. (2014) 'The long-term effects of building strong families: a program for unmarried parents', *Journal of Marriage and Family*, 76: 446–63.

3

RESPECTFUL RELATIONSHIPS EDUCATION

A case study of working in schools

Debbie Ollis and Suzanne Dyson

Introduction

> One in five young Australians believe there are circumstances in which women bear part of the responsibility for sexual assault and nearly half (46%) agree that tracking a partner by electronic means without consent is acceptable.
>
> *(Harris et al. 2015: 41)*

Gender-based violence (GBV) is a persistent social problem that is serious, prevalent and preventable. While both women and men can be victims of GBV, the vast majority of those who are affected are women. Globally, almost one third of women have experienced physical and/or sexual intimate partner violence and 7 per cent have been sexually assaulted by someone other than a partner (García-Moreno et al. 2013). In Australia nearly one in three women over the age of 15 years report being subjected to violence at some time and one in five have experienced sexual violence from a male partner or stranger (National Council to Reduce Violence against Women and their Children 2009). With recognition of the scope and impact of GBV on individuals, families and communities, prevention has become a priority. To prevent GBV it is important to understand the factors that lead some men to believe it is acceptable to use violence or abuse in their intimate relationships or with strangers. It is accepted that while individual psychological issues or socioeconomic conditions may be contributing factors, the most compelling evidence for a cause points to an association between GBV and the systemic inequalities rooted in structural power imbalances between men and women which reinforce the sense of entitlement referred to in the introductory quote (Dyson 2014; UN Women 2015).

Because GBV is so deeply entrenched, prevention efforts focus on settings where individuals live, work and play, and particular emphasis has been given to schools, where young people can be engaged in education programmes that can influence long-term attitude and behaviour change and provide some hope of changing the attitudes reflected in the most recent survey of young people's attitudes referred to in the opening quote. Despite this, research has demonstrated a paucity of evidence concerning prevention education programmes with young people that demonstrate that they actually address the predisposing factors that can lead to GBV (gender inequity and violence-supportive attitudes) or disrupt potentially violent behaviour (Tharp et al. 2011). This lack of evidence may be due to poorly designed research and evaluation; for example, some education programme evaluations that claim behavioural changes are based on self-reporting by participants and do not include long-term follow-up (Foubert et al. 2010; Fox et al. 2014; Tutty 2011).

Schools can be sites where rigid gender norms dominate and violence-supportive attitudes and behaviours thrive (Dyson 2014). For example, one study in the US reported that one in seven teenage boys think it is acceptable to force girls who flirt with them to have sex (McCauley et al. 2013). Ten per cent of Canadian teenagers report being physically hurt by their intimate partners (Tutty 2011). Another 2013 study found that 45 per cent of students who had been in dating relationships had experienced violence and 25 per cent had perpetrated it (Fox et al. 2014). A 2013 national survey of secondary students in Australia reported that 28 per cent of young women and 20 per cent of young men in years 10, 11 and 12 had experienced unwanted sex. Students cited being too drunk or pressure from their partner as the most common reasons for this (Mitchell et al. 2013).

Gender normative attitudes that reinforced hegemonic masculinity have been associated with an acceptance of violence (Sundaram 2013). Conversely gender equitable attitudes (equitable power relationships in relationships) have been found to be negatively associated with relationship violence (McCauley et al. 2013). The capacity of schools as a setting to address attitude and behaviour change is recognised internationally (Gleeson et al. 2015). The evidence suggests that effective prevention education programmes must be comprehensive and challenge the attitudes and behaviours that are violence-supportive, change the structural supports that maintain gender inequity, and use a comprehensive, multi-level, integrated approach (UN Women 2015). They should also use a whole-school approach that not only focuses on student learning, behaviour and wellbeing, but implements consistent strategies across the entire school and school community (Dyson 2009; Maxwell and Aggleton 2014; Ollis 2013; Sundaram et al. 2016). While departments of education and education experts almost universally advocate such an approach, anecdotally many schools find it difficult to implement and for some a whole-school approach represents an additional layer of work in an already crowded and time-poor curriculum (Kearney et al. 2016). In the main, secondary schools include a focus on respectful relationships in the sexuality education curriculum. However, young people report dissatisfaction with these programmes, particularly in relation to the lack of content concerning relationships, negotiating consent and sexual violence (Carmody and Willis 2006; Johnson et al. 2016).

Respectful Relationships Education in Schools project

This chapter will focus on the findings of research undertaken to assist the evaluation of a government-funded GBV prevention programme carried out in a diverse range of 19 secondary schools in Victoria, Australia in 2015. The programme, known as *Respectful Relationships Education in Schools (RREiS)*, advocates using a whole-school approach that focuses on the school's ethos and environment, its policies, and its wider community.

Curriculum, teaching and learning aspects of the programme were supported by the introduction of resources, including a curriculum resource called *Building Respectful Relationships: stepping out against gender-based violence (BRR)* (Department of Education and Early Childhood Development 2014) and associated teaching and learning resources. The curriculum and resources, which were developed by Ollis, aim to assist young people to make sense of gender (in)equity, power and violence by examining the discourses made available to them through a range of gendered subject positions, language and social institutions.

To focus on the issues of gender and power at the root of GBV (Connell 2002; Weedon 1999) a feminist, post-structural theoretical framework was used in the development of the *BRR* curriculum, an approach that has been widely supported by other scholars (e.g. Martino and Kehler 2007; Maxwell and Aggleton 2010; Renold 2006). *BRR* draws in part on Carmody's (2005) 'Sexual Ethics' framework, which is based on the premise that being a sexually ethical person is about the relationship one has with one's self and others, or care of self (Foucault 1980), which is intimately connected with relations of power and knowledge. The link between ethics, self and agency is a key focus in the materials which start from the assumption that sexuality is positive, and link information and critical thinking with empowerment, choice and inclusion of diversity.

The *BRR* resource includes two units of work, one designed for grade eight (12–13 years old) and one designed for grade nine students (14–15 years old). The grade eight unit, *Gender, Respect and Relationships*, is designed to provide the grounding to examine issues in GBV such as sexual assault, domestic violence and homophobia. The unit aims to explore and develop a common understanding of gender, relationships and respect. Students examine the implications for relationships of gendered assumptions around masculinities, femininities and sexualities, and begin to develop skills in communication, negotiation, deconstruction, reconstruction, reflection and media literacy (Department of Education and Early Childhood Development 2014). The grade nine unit, *The Power Connection*, is built on concepts covered in grade eight and aims to explore the nature of GBV and the implications for respectful and ethical practice. It specifically explores domestic violence and sexual assault in the context of power, social and institutional structure, and young people's lives. This unit takes a broad view of violence, covering the physical, emotional, social and economic implications of GBV, including homophobia. In addition, it is designed to assist students to understand the nature of consent and respect, and develop skills to take individual and collective action and responsibility for self and others (Department of Education and Early Childhood Development 2014). Students engaged with the curriculum over one to two school terms (10–20 weeks) depending on the curriculum structure of the school. Professional development was made available to most teachers prior to the teaching programme.

In the following sections of this chapter we discuss the *RREiS* evaluation methodology and the findings, which include three key themes: evaluation findings for students, for school staff and overall outcomes of the programme from the perspective of members of the school community over the course of one year. Finally, the discussion section will focus on the implications of the findings for teaching respectful relationship education in schools.

Methodology

The evaluation used mixed qualitative and quantitative methods; however, this chapter draws only on the qualitative data. Interviews and focus groups were conducted with a sample of students and teachers from nine schools involved in the *RREiS* project (approximately half of the schools involved in the project) (see Kearny et al. 2016 for more information on the project). Data were collected from 30 focus group interviews, including with students who were recipients of the education (71 grade eight/nine students, 30 females and 41 males), teaching staff involved in teaching the curriculum (43 participants, 25 females and 18 males) and leadership teams which generally consisted of the principal, assistant principal, student wellbeing coordinator and other school leadership positions depending on the size of the school (38 participants, 24 females and 14 males). Interviews were conducted during October and November 2015. Interview questions focused on understandings of the key concepts in the curriculum, the experience of being taught or teaching the curriculum, observed changes in behaviour, the impact on the culture of the school, attitudes to gender-based violence, and key barriers and enablers to implementation in the classroom. Data were analysed thematically and the research received approval from both the Deakin University Human Ethics Committee and the Victorian Department of Education. The research was funded by the Victorian government and coordinated by Our Watch.

Findings: students

Understanding key concepts

Following participation in the classroom programme students demonstrated a clear understanding about gender, gender equality and violence. For example, one young man explained, 'Gender is not what sex you are but what you want to be,' and another stated, 'People think that sexual assault is about sex but it's about power.' Power, a sense of entitlement and hierarchies were mentioned by a number of students. Some attempted to articulate the difference between equity and equality; for example, one young man explained:

> Equity, kind of . . . equality is like if you had two candies, you'd give one to one person and one to the other. But then equity is like – if you have two candies, I don't need any candy and that person needs it, you give it all to them.

Quotes such as this demonstrate that students who participated in *RREiS* were processing the complexity of gender relations, equity and inequality. Students were also able to make the connection between these concepts and GBV. One explained:

> We learnt about how men are always told that they have to be more dominant and they can't express their emotions and so they would feel like they would have to not tell anyone because people would see them as weak. We've been brought up [with the idea that] males must be seen as manly and females as seen as females, which is totally wrong but that's just how we see it as a society . . . males are seen as stronger than females. I guess in families men could take charge and boss around the wife and things like that. That could cause domestic violence when the woman tries to stand against it.

There was also evidence that students, particularly boys, saw the importance of the respectful relationships education for future gender equality. As one male student commented:

> I think it's a good idea to have this sort of programme in more schools. It'll stop the system, like boys growing up thinking that they should be the more dominant person in the relationship and learning this now might stop that and make it less of a problem, gender equality.

Although this chapter is concerned with the qualitative data collected by Ollis in 2015, as part of the larger evaluation of the *RREiS* project, students' knowledge of, attitudes towards and confidence in discussing issues of domestic violence, gender equality and respectful relationships was also mirrored in the results of the student surveys. There was improvement across *all* 24 survey questions that were used to collect quantitative data by the project team:
    For example, the proportion of students who felt that

> *'slapping or pushing a partner to cause harm or fear'* was a form of domestic violence increased from 70% of students in the baseline survey to 80% of students in the follow-up survey.
>
> (Kearney et al. 2016: 7)

Understanding GBV and family violence

Most students had a clear understanding about the gendered nature of violence against women, explaining that the majority of perpetrators 'tend to be men' although they were surprised by the statistics. They understood that GBV could take many forms; one group of students explained:

> Family violence is any sort of emotional, physical violence within your family . . . Financial as well . . . Sexual . . . Emotional . . . With any relation whatsoever, including your boyfriend or girlfriend . . . It can happen with [sic] just once and that still counts as well.

Learning about sexual consent was another important focus for both students and teachers, in particular legal issues, for example:

> I really like the way how they highlighted that you need consent before doing anything. You can't force anything on anyone, unless you have consent, don't do it, it's just you need[,] both people need to reach an agreement.

Respect and respectful relationships

In focus groups students maintained that the *RREiS* programme had positively changed their own and others' behaviour and understanding of respectful relationships. For example, one student explained that students who would normally make sexist or homophobic comments were being silenced and were 'not going to say [things like] that even if they thought it'. There were a number of examples of personal change. One young woman explained:

> [I've come to understand] what you want in a relationship and what you don't want. To know how to have a respectful relationship . . . it's very hard to open up in an abusive relationship, as I've been in one myself.

Some of the young men recognised the potential impact of their own behaviours. One explained:

> Before respectful relationships I was a very, very, very angry person. I had a massive temper. But after learning a few things about respectful relationships and everything like that I've kind of calmed down.

Both teachers and students enjoyed the activity-based teaching and learning approach. A common theme in student focus groups was that the approach 'didn't force us to have an opinion, they just let us express our opinions and then taught us a few things and saw our opinions change. They never forced anything for us to believe.'

Findings: teaching staff

Several key themes emerged from discussions with teachers in relation to teaching and learning, including the challenges involved in using a whole-school approach in busy school settings, of connecting sexuality education with respectful relationships education, and the importance of professional development and support for staff who teach respectful relationships.

From grand ideas to small changes

Schools opted-in to participate in *RREiS* and a key driver for participation was a belief in these schools that students would benefit from a curriculum on respectful relationships. Teaching staff began the project with a commitment to and passion for whole-school change. Nonetheless, structural constraints and barriers within the school combined with the demands of teaching made it difficult for teachers to work beyond their individual classrooms, as one female teacher articulated:

> We walked in really passionate and really excited and then . . . 'no it's not your job to change policy' . . . I just felt really deflated. Then we had welfare saying yes we'll come on board and that sort of fell apart too. I started to feel really bashed. In the end we just said you know what? Let's just teach the kids. I know it's supposed to be about the culture of the school, but let's just worry about hitting the kids hard with this stuff and that hopefully we will see some change. We just – yeah from grand ideas to small changes.

There were significant variations in the curriculum approach taken in different schools. Although the content was covered in health and sexuality education and overwhelmingly taught by health and physical education teachers, there were examples of other staff being required to teach at the last minute due to staff shortages. This included an English teacher, school nurse and two chaplains, none of whom had participated in the professional learning workshop. These inconsistencies resulted in the programme being taught by staff members who lacked understanding about the curriculum and its content. One outcome of this related to misinformation about men as victims of GBV, which resulted in confusion for the students (discussed in more depth below).

Time was another challenge for teachers – some schools had four sessions a week while others had only one. This impacted on what could be covered and the depth with which teachers were able to cover the content. A number of teachers were frustrated with the demands of the curriculum in the time available. They felt they had to 'skim important issues' and had little time to diverge when needed. To overcome these limitations some schools developed innovative approaches. In one school where time was extremely limited they bookended a weekly session with two half days, one at the beginning of the term and the other at the end. In another, the school embedded the curriculum into a four-day intensive 'challenge programme'.

Despite the challenges, teachers demonstrated skill in modifying, adapting and extending the curriculum in line with student needs and the school's ethos.

For example, a group of teachers modified *BRR* to address low literacy levels and engage their students in exploring the connection between behaviour, language and gender-based violence by creating games and observing behaviour as the games progressed. They explained:

> we finished that about 30 minutes into the session and we started writing up on the board the dialogue that we'd had between the kids; 'oh my god you throw like a girl' and all that kind of stuff.

Make sure you've got the right resources

Teachers were adamant that having resources that are well-planned, easy to deliver and contain useful tools was critical. They argued that having activities that are fun, interesting and interactive, that prompt discussion about taboo topics and increase both student and teacher knowledge, built their confidence and made the teaching experience positive and enjoyable. For example:

> You've just got to make sure you've got the right resources and you can just sort of run in there, you feel confident about what you're actually going to teach. But having this sort of stuff is pretty good too.

A number of teachers raised the importance of students having a background in sexuality education before the *BRR* curriculum. Schools which implemented *BRR* prior to their sexuality education curriculum felt that students struggled with issues such as sexual assault, for example:

> The heavy stuff was more of the sexual, not so much the gender, like the gender stereotypes, like they got through okay but it was more of the sexuality I think that, because we hadn't done the sex-ed first whereas I think the combination might work better.

Professional development and support

Both teachers and school leadership teams acknowledged the critical role of professional development as a key factor for teaching the curriculum. Professional development built confidence, awareness, knowledge and commitment to the prevention of violence against women. It provided the opportunity both to develop skills and pedagogical approaches that engaged the students in a safe learning environment and to become familiar with the *BRR*. They used words such as 'motivating' and 'fantastic'. One expanded:

> I didn't know how to teach about domestic violence. Like unless I had a bit of background in health, like there's just no way. I wouldn't feel comfortable at all.

Not all teachers had the opportunity to attend the professional learning, which had negative implications for how the curriculum was taught:

> I think it might fall over if no one's doing the training because it'll come back to me having to sit down with a staff member and I'm not *au fait* with everything to be able to train them as well. Then it's done hodgepodge and it's not done with the best intentions.

In schools where teachers were unable to participate in the two-day workshop, teachers found the experience more challenging and struggled with handling student questions and divergent opinions. Some teachers who did not attend the professional development did not understand the project aims or the nature and extent of violence against women. These teachers gave students different messages to those communicated in the professional development and in the curriculum. One male teacher who had not done the professional development explained: 'a lot of [the kids] have that misconception, that domestic violence is mainly women'. While men can be victims of family violence, as discussed in the introduction, the vast majority of those who experience GBV are indeed women. This teacher's misinformation contradicted the curriculum and led to confusion for the students in his classes. While many students were able to articulate the reality of violence against women and the nature and extent of family violence, some also maintained that they had learned 'that we need to talk about how the women can be violent to men'.

Another key factor for teachers delivering the BRR programme was leadership support. There were a number of examples in which teachers felt that they did not receive this, which impacted negatively on how effectively they could implement the programme. In addition to leadership support, schools valued the idea of support from external agencies, although very few actually used these resources.

Findings: moving towards whole-school change

The major outcome of the BRR programme for students, teachers and school leaders concerns changes in the school culture and changes in student behaviour. In the words of one assistant principal: 'after the respectful relationships, the feedback I got from two of the teachers was mind blowing how they had changed . . . yeah, big change'.

Many of the students said that they did not know what a respectful relationship was prior to the programme; they referred to the importance of 'just learning what respect is and what people expect for respect'. There were also many examples of schools using the respectful relationship teaching and learning as a framework to build respectful behaviour across the school. One teacher explained:

> I had a PE class yesterday and a kid said, 'oh you throw like a girl'. I was like 'excuse me?' He was like, 'oh sorry, sorry'. Like they know straight away now. Whereas I think they didn't know that before.

This extended across the entire school. The leadership teams were using this in a disciplinary sense to remind students and staff of the need to 'name it' outside the classroom as well as within. Teachers used the approach to guide the classroom environment and students used it to demand respectful practices from other students and the school. Teachers also felt that it had given girls in particular the confidence to report sexist and disrespectful behaviours. They also referred to the positive impact of the programme on student participation. One explained, 'I had a few students that never put their hand up in any other subject. [But] they were really keen to share their views [in *BRR*].' Another said:

> I've got girls that have been in relationships and it's all clicking. They're like he wouldn't let me see my friends. It's those aha moments. The kids are really good at saying yeah I get what you're talking about now because it's clicked. I think that's why I really do love this programme. I think it's brilliant.

Another example of the impact of the programme on individual students was articulated by a teacher who explained that he had a male student with a history of violence who asked if he could leave the room during one of the sessions. The teacher found the student sobbing outside:

> I said to him, 'Where's this coming from?' and he goes – he couldn't even speak. I said, 'Is this reflection?' He goes 'yeah like' – so he was actually reflecting on what he does and how that impacts on others . . . There's been massive improvement, even since then. Like now he wants to go and get help outside school because he doesn't want to be like that.

Discussion: implications for practice in schools

The findings from this research suggest that the *BRR* resources and teaching approaches have assisted students in grade eight and nine to develop an understanding of respectful relationships. Students demonstrated high levels of understanding about the key concepts and aims of the curriculum, and their knowledge about violence against women exceeded expectations. The evaluation of the earlier trial of the *BRR* resource in 2010 (see Ollis 2014) found that students struggled with the concept of power and its relationship to gender and violence. This was not the case in the *RREiS* programme. The key differences in the two projects help to explain this and provide some direction for future implementation.

To begin with, schools and teachers elected to be part of the *RREiS* project while in 2010 the schools involved were required by the education authority to participate. This has enormous implications for the way schools engage with projects designed to bring about some type of cultural change. As other health research has shown, there must be readiness for change (Gardner and Ollis 2015) which involves building awareness, commitment and motivation by the entire school community (Samdal and Rowling 2011). Professional learning is needed to build the knowledge and comfort of the teachers to teach it (Ollis 2013), and resources must be made available to support teachers to plan and implement education programmes within a context of support. Schools in *RREiS* had strong leadership teams that demonstrated both a top-down and bottom-up approach, a factor identified in the literature as important in building commitment and ensuring a commitment from all sections of the school (Dooris 2009; Dyson 2008).

The curriculum was implemented overwhelmingly in the health and physical discipline context, using pedagogies familiar to anyone teaching health and sexuality education. In 2010 this was not the case and teachers from other disciplines struggled with the unfamiliar nature of the activity-based approach or dealing with the sensitive issues (Ollis 2014). The positive response from the health and physical education teachers involved in teaching *BRR* in 2015 indicates the need to ensure that respectful relationships education is integrated into the existing health education curriculum as outlined in the new Australian Curriculum (ACARA 2013) rather than providing a stand-alone programme delivered by outside agencies, characteristic of current approaches in many countries (Stanley et al. 2015).

The ability of schools and teachers to tailor the curriculum to individual school structures and student needs, such as intensive models and team teaching, increased the success of the classroom programme by providing a sustainable context for future work. In addition, the professional development and ongoing support provided as part of the programme and the additional resources, debriefing and ongoing training were not available in 2010. Moreover, *BRR* was updated in 2011 and a professional learning programme developed in 2012 using the findings and results of the 2010 trial. Following the 2010 evaluation, the limitations of the *BRR* resource were addressed and the findings of the *RREiS* evaluation demonstrate that these limitations were overcome.

The powerful impact of the teaching and learning experience was the increase in student recognition and understanding of respect and respectful relationships. This is an encouraging finding for the prevention of GBV. It indicates that an explicit focus on gender equity and respectful relationships can work to raise students' awareness about not only the nature and extent of GBV but also how this is relevant to their own lived experience. It is clear from this research that concerns about protecting the innocence of young people, or demonising men, often cited as reasons for not doing this work, are unfounded (Allen 2011). Both young men and young women in this study continually talked about the importance of the education for their futures as respected and respectful adults. This is consistent with the most recent Australian research with 2,500 young people about what they want to learn about in sexuality and relationships education programmes (Johnson et al. 2016).

The use of the formal curriculum to support a broader policy and practice approach to student management and respectful practices is another promising finding from this research. School leaders and teachers constantly referred to the positive impact of reminding students about what they were learning about respect and how this differed to their current behaviour. It also appeared to give students confidence to report disrespectful practices without fear of reprisal. Hillier et al. (2010) found a similar result in their study of same-sex attracted young people in schools. Making policy visible to young people helps them to feel safe and respected.

There are a number of challenges for schools as they educate young people about respectful relationships, gender-based violence and violence against women: building teacher confidence, knowledge and comfort, including pre-service teacher education; integrating the curriculum into existing and sustainable structures; resources to enable planning and professional development and time to build relationships with the community that support schools and students. Even so, this research has shown that, contrary to espoused beliefs – evident in popular media over the past few months (Latham 2016) – young people are able and comfortable to position this education in a feminist and gender equity framework. There was no opposition from students, only recognition and a desire to change things. The more difficult task was implementing whole-school approaches that can support and complement the work of the classroom teacher. Moving forward, this is the challenge.

Acknowledgements

We would like to acknowledge the work of the Our Watch Evaluation team, Sarah Kearney and Loksee Leung who coordinated the *RREiS* research project on which the data in this chapter is based.

References

ACARA (Australian Curriculum and Assessment Authority) (2013) *Draft F–10 Australian Curriculum: health and physical education consultation report*, Sydney: Australian Curriculum, Assessment and Reporting Authority.

Allen, L. (2011) *Young People and Sexuality Education: rethinking key debates*, Basingstoke: Palgrave Macmillan.

Carmody, M. (2005) 'Ethical erotics: reconceptualizing anti-rape education', *Sexualities*, 8: 465–80.

Carmody, M. and Willis, K. (2006) *Developing Ethical Sexual Lives: young people, sex and sexual assault prevention*, Sydney: University of Western Sydney, NSW Rape Crisis Centre.

Connell, R. (2002) *Gender*, Cambridge: Polity Press.

Department of Education and Early Childhood Development (2014) *Building Respectful Relationships: stepping out against gender based violence*, Melbourne: Government of Victoria, Department of Education and Early Childhood Development.

Dooris, M. (2009) 'Holistic and sustainable health improvement: the contribution of the settings-based approach to health promotion', *Perspectives in Public Health*, 129: 29–36.

Dyson, S. (2008) *Catching on Everywhere: evaluation of a whole school sexuality education project in 50 Victorian schools*. Online. Available at www.eduweb.vic.gov.au/edulibrary/public/teachlearn/student/coeverywherept1.pdf (accessed 16 March 2017).

Dyson, S. (2009) 'Girls and well-being: why educators should promote respectful relationships in school programs', *Redress: Journal of the Association of Women Educators*, 18(1): 8–13.

Dyson, S. (2014) *Health and the Primary Prevention of Violence against Women, Position Paper 2014*, Drysdale, Victoria: Australian Women's Health Network.

Foubert, J.D., Godin, E.E. and Tatum, J.L. (2010) 'In their own words: sophomore college men describe attitude and behavior changes resulting from a rape prevention program 2 years after their participation', *Journal of Interpersonal Violence*, 25: 2237–57.

Foucault, M. (1980) *Power/Knowledge*, New York: Harvester Press.

Fox, C., Corr, M. and Gadd, D. (2014) 'Young teenagers' experience of domestic abuse', *Journal of Youth Studies*, 17: 510–26.

García-Moreno, C., Pallitto, C., Devries, K., Stöckl, H., Watts, C. and Abrahams, N. (2013) *Global and Regional Estimates of Violence against Women: prevalence and health effects of intimate partner violence and non-partner sexual violence*, Geneva: World Health Organization. Online. Available at http://apps.who.int/iris/bitstream/10665/85239/1/9789241564625_eng.pdf (accessed 18 May 2016).

Gardner, B. and Ollis, D. (2015) '"Change in schools it's more like sort of turning an oil tanker": creating readiness for health promoting schools', *Health Research*, 115: 377–91.

Gleeson, C., Kearney S., Leung, L. and Brislane, J. (2015) *Respectful Relationships Education in Schools: evidence paper*. Online. Available at www.ourwatch.org.au/getmedia/4a61e08b-c958-40bc-8e02-30fde5f66a25/Evidence-paper-respectful-relationships-education-AAupdated.pdf.aspx (accessed 2 February 2016).

Harris, A., Honey, N., Webster, K., Diemer, K. and Polito, V. (2015) *Young Australians' Attitudes to Violence against Women: findings from the 2013 National Community Attitudes towards Violence against Women Survey for respondents 16–24 years*, Melbourne: Victorian Health Promotion Foundation.

Hillier, L., Jones, T., Monagle, M., Overton, N., Gahan, L., Blackman, J. and Mitchell, A. (2010) *Writing Themselves in 3: the third national study of the sexual health and wellbeing of same-sex attracted and gender questioning young people*, Monograph series no. 78, Melbourne: The Australian Research Centre in Sex, Health and Society, La Trobe University.

Johnson, B., Harrison, L., Ollis, D., Arnold, P., Flentje, J. and Bartholomeaus, C. (2016) *Engaging Young People in Sexuality Education, Report of Phase 1*, Adelaide: University of South Australia.

Kearney, S., Gleeson, C., Leung, L., Ollis, D. and, Joyce, A. (2016) *Respectful Relationships Education in Schools: the beginnings of change – research report*, Melbourne: Our Watch.

Latham, M. (2016) 'Neo-Marxist feminists send a neutered Trojan Horse into schools to re-engineer our children's sexuality and social values', *Daily Telegraph*, 26 April 2016.

McCauley, H., Tancredi, D., Silverman, J.G., Decker, M., Austin, S.B. and Jones, K. (2013) 'Gender-equitable attitudes, bystander behavior, and recent abuse perpetration against heterosexual dating partners of male high school athletes', *American Journal of Public Health*, 103: 1882–7.

Martino, W. and Kehler, M. (2007) 'Gender-based literacy reform: a question of challenging or recuperating gender binaries', *Canadian Journal of Education/Revue Canadienne de l'éducation*, 30: 406–31.

Maxwell, C. and Aggleton, P. (2010) 'The bubble of privilege: young, privately educated women talk about social class', *British Journal of Sociology of Education*, 31: 3–15.

Maxwell, C. and Aggleton, P. (2014) 'Preventing violence against women and girls: utilising a "whole school approach"', in J. Ellis and R.K. Thiara (eds) *Preventing Violence against Women and Girls: educational work with children and young people*, Bristol: Policy Press.

Mitchell, A., Kent, P., Heywood, W., Blackman, P. and Pitts, M. (2013) *5th National Survey of Australian Secondary Students and Sexual Health*, Melbourne: Australian Research Centre in Sex, Health and Society, La Trobe University.

National Council to Reduce Violence against Women and their Children (2009) *A Time for Action: the National Council's plan for Australia to reduce violence against women and their children, 2009–2021*, Canberra: Commonwealth of Australia.

Ollis, D. (2013) 'Planning and delivering interventions to promote gender and sexuality', in I. Rivers and N. Duncan (eds) *Bullying: experiences and discourses of sexuality and gender*, London: Routledge.

Ollis, D. (2014) 'The role of teachers in delivering education about respectful relationships: exploring teacher and student perspectives', *Health Education Research*, 29: 702–13.

Renold, E. (2006) '"They won't let us play ... unless you're going out with one of them": girls, boys and Butler's "heterosexual matrix" in the primary years', *British Journal of Sociology of Education*, 27: 489–509.

Samdal, O. and Rowling, L. (2011) 'Theoretical and empirical base for implementation components of health-promoting schools', *Health Education*, 111: 367–90.

Stanley, N., Ellis, J., Farrelly, N., Hollinghurst, S., Bailey, S. and Downe, S. (2015) 'Preventing domestic abuse for children and young people (PEACH): a mixed knowledge scoping review', *Public Health Research*, 3(7). Online. Available at http://dx.doi.org/10.3310/phr03070 (accessed 1 March 2017).

Sundaram, V. (2013) 'Violence as understandable, deserved or unacceptable? Listening for gender in teenagers' talk about violence', *Gender and Education*, 25: 889–906.

Sundaram, V., Maxwell, C. and Ollis, D. (2016) 'Where does violence against women and girls work fit in? Exploring spaces for challenging violence within a sex-positive framework in schools', in V. Sundaram and H. Sauntson (eds) *Global Perspectives and Key Debates in Sex and Relationships Education: addressing issues of gender, sexuality, plurality and power*, Basingstoke: Palgrave MacMillan.

Tharp, A., De Gue, S., Lang, K., Valle, L., Massetti, G., Holt, M. and Matjasko, J. (2011) 'Commentary on Foubert, Godin and Tatum (2010): the evolution of sexual violence prevention and the urgency for effectiveness', *Journal of Interpersonal Violence*, 26: 3383–92.

Tutty, L. (2011) *Healthy Relationships Preventing Teen Dating Violence: an evaluation of the Teen Violence Prevention Program*, Toronto: Canadian Women's Foundation.

UN Women (2015) *A Framework to Underpin Action to Prevent Violence Against Women*. Online. Available at www2.unwomen.org/~/media/headquarters/attachments/sections/library/publications/2015/prevention_framework_unwomen_nov2015.pdf?v=1andd=20151124T225223 (accessed 3 February 2016).

Weedon, C. (1999) *Feminism, Theory and the Politics of Difference*, Oxford: Blackwell Publishers.

4

MEETING ADOLESCENTS 'WHERE THEY'RE AT'

The use of technology to prevent violence and abuse in adolescent romantic relationships

Erica Bowen and Emma Sorbring

Introduction

Adolescent dating violence (ADV) is a public health concern which carries with it a substantial disease burden. Consequences of ADV span physical and mental health and also lead to adult relationship difficulties, disrupted education and poor lifetime attainment. Primary prevention programmes offered to school children typically elicit modest effects. Consequently, there may be some potential in developing alternative and innovative methods of primary prevention. Drawing on the EU-funded 'Changing Attitudes towards dating Violence in Adolescence (CAVA)' project this chapter examines the potential of using computer technology, and more specifically, digital or 'serious' games in the development of primary prevention approaches.

Adolescent dating violence

Research shows that risk for violence and abuse within intimate relationships is greatest in adolescence and typically reduces during early adulthood (Johnson et al. 2015). Adolescent dating violence typically comprises a range of behaviours including verbal, psychological, physical and sexual aggression (Bowen and Walker 2015). A comprehensive international (Europe and North America) review of the prevalence of such violence by Leen et al. (2013) found that rates of physical ADV ranged between 10 and 20 per cent of the general population samples with rates similar for boys and girls. Great variability was reported in rates of sexual ADV (from 1.2 per cent to 75 per cent), although the inclusion of verbal sexual aggression may account for some of the higher rates found. Across studies psychological ADV was more prevalent than physical and sexual ADV, and prevalence rates were similar for girls and boys in the majority of the reported studies across all forms of

ADV (Leen et al. 2013). Qualitative studies indicate, however, that even when similar rates of victimisation are identified for boys and girls, girls are more negatively impacted by their experiences (e.g. Barter et al. 2009). The use of new communication technologies by adolescents has also facilitated ADV and, as a recent review has illustrated, the rates of technology-assisted ADV experienced by adolescents are concerning (Stonard et al. 2015).

ADV is associated with a range of negative outcomes including lower self-esteem and negative self-concept, anxiety and depressive symptoms, reported suicidal thoughts and attempts, substance use and alcohol abuse (Temple et al. 2013), unwanted pregnancy and sexually transmitted infections (Shorey et al. 2015), and eating disorders (Exner-Cortens et al. 2013). There is also some evidence that ADV disrupts education and educational attainment (Bowen and Walker 2015). Consequently, there is a clear need to educate adolescents about ADV so that they can recognise abuse and violence within their own relationships and those of their peers, and learn how to deal with the situation should it arise. Indeed, school-based primary prevention programmes have been found to be effective in the prevention of violence within adolescent intimate relationships although by their nature such interventions typically produce modest effects (Wolfe et al. 2009).

Why consider the use of digital games?

The use of communication technology and digital technologies is particularly salient during adolescence. This age group is more likely to use the internet, own gaming devices, go online wirelessly (via laptops and phones), use social networking sites, and download and use apps on their phones. The rise in their popularity has raised questions about the potential pedagogical benefits of incorporating digital media in the classroom (Smetana and Bell 2012).

Individuals vary in relation to their preferred mode of learning, and consequently relying on print materials that are typically used in classroom teaching may not meet the diverse needs of all the children in a classroom (Shin et al. 2012). Therefore, educational material that appeals to multiple modes of learning, e.g. text, picture, video, animation and audio, may address the different abilities, needs and interests of the individual learner in the classroom (Rose et al. 2005). Digital or 'serious' games can also encourage children to explore new ideas (Hoffmann 2009). By definition, a serious game (SG) is an application developed that uses technologies from computer games that serve purposes other than pure entertainment (Arnab et al. 2013). Modern educational SGs are thought to be effective teaching tools for enhancing learning as they use action, encourage motivation, accommodate multiple learning styles, reinforce skills, and provide an interactive and decision-making context (Charles and McAlister 2004). In addition, SGs allow students to gather new information and align this with previous knowledge and experience as well as enabling them to be active in the control of their learning in an individualised way (Dempsey et al. 2002).

Researchers agree that SGs have all the attributes to be effective learning plat-forms (Connolly et al. 2012), and there is evidence of their effectiveness in the context of maths (Ke 2013), science (Sung and Hwang 2013) and geography (Virvou and Katsionis 2008) education. Evidence suggests that games promote active learning (Mellecker et al. 2013); curiosity, positive learning attitudes and motivation (Kovačević et al. 2013); improvement in learning achievement and self-efficacy (Sung and Hwang 2013); learning of high-level or complex skills (Hainey et al. 2011); and engagement with curriculum content (Walsh 2010).

A small corpus of literature also indicates that SGs are now being used to teach more sensitive, non-STEM (science, technology, engineering and mathematics) subjects, including healthy eating (Majumdar et al. 2012), reducing illegal substance abuse (Gamberini et al. 2009), diabetes (Thompson et al. 2010), and relationship and sex education (RSE) (Arnab et al. 2013; Gilliam et al. 2016). Arnab et al. (2013) reported positive outcomes using a game-based approach intervention designed to teach adolescents how to identify and prevent coercion in their relationships. In a cluster randomised controlled trial, engaging with the game was found to lead to greater self-reported confidence to recognise coercion, knowledge of how to say no to others, and understanding of personal risk. The authors concluded that there is a real advantage for pedagogy-driven game-based approaches to be utilised when delivering RSE in the classroom. In a more recent study Gilliam et al. (2016) report on the co-created game developed to facilitate discussion and reporting of sexual violence by school children. It was found that the game led to the initiation of con-versations about sexual violence in nearly all children at follow up, and improved knowledge and understanding of the topic. This supports the use of SG when dealing with non-STEM subjects, particularly those of a sensitive nature. However, although quantitative outcomes were positive, it was not clear what it was about the game environment that could have led to such outcomes. Taken together this evidence indicates that there could be some potential in developing a serious game based intervention for ADV.

Developing a serious game to prevent ADV

Between 2011 and 2013 the first author held an EU Daphne III funded transna-tional action grant to develop a serious game to raise awareness of dating violence and its risk factors and improve help-seeking among young people aged 12–16 years. Project partners were recruited from the UK, Sweden, Belgium and Germany. The vision was to develop a free-to-use tool that teachers could implement within the school curriculum that would help educate young people on this topic in a way that was acceptable to all involved. Although most schools do include an ele-ment of relationship education in their teaching, this varies from school to school in terms of content, style and time spent, and is very dependent on the skill set, ability and interest of individual teachers, so using digital resources enables consistency of delivery (Arnab et al. 2013). The role of education in combating violence against women is clearly stated in the *European Convention on Preventing and Combating Violence against Women and Domestic Violence* (Council of Europe 2011) and schools are identified as an important avenue through which young people can be educated about the nature of, and factors associated with, violence and abuse in relationships.

Green Acres High

Green Acres High is an SG based on Adobe Flash that runs in an internet browser compatible with Internet Explorer (v 8.4 onwards) and comprises five, fully computer-mediated 'lessons', each of which concentrates on a different aspect of learning about dating violence. The sessions focused on defining healthy relationships, identifying risk factors for abuse, characteristics of abusive relationships, conflict resolution and safe help-seeking. Decisions about content were taken through two phases of research: (i) a literature review to determine what is known about the prevalence of dating violence in Europe, dynamic risk factors for adolescent dating violence, and effective primary intervention approaches (Leen et al. 2013); and (ii) a focus group study conducted with 86 young people (50 females, 36 males) aged 12–16 years across the four partner countries (Bowen et al. 2013). The premise of both aspects of the research was to determine what we know from a European perspective about the nature of dating violence, effective primary intervention approaches, and also attitudes about dating violence held by European adolescents. This last point was of particular relevance given the findings from the first piece of research that attitudes towards dating violence have been the most widely empirically supported dynamic risk factor for engaging in dating violence behaviours (Bowen et al. 2013). The focus group study was a replication of the only other qualitative investigation of adolescent attitudes, which had been conducted in Canada (Sears et al. 2006).

Our focus group data highlighted that European adolescents share many of the same attitudes towards dating violence that have been reported in North American groups. Specifically, although adolescents generally did not endorse the use of violence, there were several clear contexts in which violence was not only permitted, but also in some instances expected. These included violence as a one-off, violence in retaliation for being cheated on, violence in the context of a joke, violence used by girls. It was also clear that adolescents upheld traditional gender-role stereotypes in relation to violence, with violence by men towards women criticised, but violence by women or girls towards men or boys viewed as not being violence. Help-seeking was also gendered whereby males would not disclose abuse because of stereotypical male identities, and because women's use of violence is less severe and not defined as violence. Decisions to seek help were also related to severity of the violence. There was a hierarchy of violent acts, with more severe acts (e.g. punching, kicking) being less acceptable, and less severe acts (e.g. pushing, slapping) being more acceptable. In addition, young people reported that if they did seek help, they would be most likely to seek it from their friends rather than from adults.

The findings from both these studies supported a case for the potential impact of a brief (five-session) classroom-based intervention on attitudes towards dating violence, at least in the short term.

A decision was taken therefore to review the content of existing classroom-based interventions as these all focus on raising awareness about the nature of violence, as well as challenging attitudes that support its use and stereotypical gender-role attitudes, and providing conflict resolution skills training and help-seeking advice. A number of manuals and toolkits were obtained including *Expect Respect* (Home Office and Women's Aid n.d.), *Save the Date* (Family Violence Project 2007) and *Healthy Relationships* (Men for Change 1994), and descriptions of key tasks were noted with regard to how they could inspire the content of the game. In conjunction with the game developers, a narrative storyline was developed within which the attitude change and/or behavioural change techniques could be implanted through interactive exercises. To ensure that the techniques employed in the game were evidence-based, a mapping exercise was undertaken through which the key techniques were identified in relation to their theory and utility using the taxonomy identified by Abraham and Michie (2008). Specific details of this process are reported in Bowen et al. (2014). The majority of attitude/behaviour change techniques adopted were based on four theories of behaviour change: socio-cognitive, information-motivation-behavioural skills model, control theory, and operant conditioning.

Pilot evaluation

We conducted a small-scale pilot qualitative evaluation using three focus groups with 13 English young people who had played the game (see Bowen et al. 2014 for details). Overall, young people found the format of using the game acceptable, and the general feedback was very positive. In fact the only negative aspects related to the technical functionality as the technology available to schools to run the game was not of a contemporary specification, which at times meant that the game was slow to load. In addition, students highlighted aspects of programmed game functionality that did not work as effectively as they could have done, specifically that more instructions were needed at times to help them navigate around the game.

When describing the positive features of the game, themes emerged around the role of experiential learning as adolescents found that a positive aspect of the game was learning through experience. Through the game the adolescents came into contact with some of the issues, decisions, factors and processes related to ADV. This made learning more of a hands-on experience. Adolescents acknowledged that learning had occurred and therefore playing the game was a positive and worthwhile experience. Specific themes were identified as learning through doing and interactive engagement, discovery through autonomy and informed choices, and transferable knowledge gathering.

Learning through doing and interactive engagement

Adolescents liked the fact that the game was interactive and that they were able to achieve specific learning goals and accomplish specific tasks within the context of a story. The adolescents identified that key to the process of learning through 'doing' was the fact that the experiences were interactive (the numerals refer to the number of the focus group, the letters to the participant):

> 1A: I think people are more likely to listen more instead of just a teacher telling you stuff; people will actually interact with the game because it's just you and a computer.

> 2A: I think the game is quite good because it's seen as a game but it's still educational and there's still the sense that it, it's quite fun because it's interactive and you get to pick where you're going and stuff.

This interaction was achieved by getting the adolescents to assume roles or participate in activities through computer-generated real-life stories and experiences, encouraging the adolescents to make and take certain decisions. This finding raises an important observation, that it is necessary to differentiate that it is not just the case that the adolescents are using e-learning content (i.e. just being given information but through a digital medium) but that they are *playing a game* (i.e. an interactive and participatory activity):

> 2E: Well because we were in that situation, in the game we were the ones giving the advice.

Part of the process involved the players not only immersing themselves in the different situations but then making decisions based on the information they had been given and were experiencing. This was discussed by two of the game-players:

> 3B: Erm, I think it was good that they included real scenarios that could happen and it made you deal with them.

> 3C: I think it was good because it showed, showed the thing from both points of view, like from the male's point of view and the female's point of view and how they're both feeling.

Discovery through autonomy and informed choices

The adolescents valued the sense of autonomy that they felt when engaging with the game. It has been suggested that if individuals discover things on their own they are then likely to remember the concepts that they are trying to learn (Kebritchi and Hirumi 2008). This discovery through exploration and making decisions themselves is discussed by one of the focus groups:

> 1A:Yeah because one thing there was a kind of counselling session and people would say this has been happening what should I do and you have different options and then you like click on an option and then it would give you points depending on how good your decisions were.

The adolescents saw the fact that they had to make decisions in the game as a positive aspect of the game. As the adolescents were autonomous as they played the game and were offered various choices that they then had to question and decipher, this meant that they engaged with the game. This process is described by one of the adolescents:

> 2B:Yeah, it [the game] gives you options. If you're just doing like a lesson of it the teacher's the one that does the speaking and you just write stuff down whereas in the game you get to choose what you want to do and you don't, nobody else can input on it it's your choice.

Overall, the benefit of this feature of the game was that the adolescents identified that this was an effective way of learning. This was noted by one of the students:

> 3C: It sort of made us understand it more because you were like put in a situation where you had to try and sort that situation out.

Transferable knowledge gathering

Another element of the experiential learning was that, through the interactive games, knowledge was gathered by the adolescents that they then felt could be used in practice in real life and on a day-to-day basis. One of the elements that the adolescents identified as being positive was that they learned how to recognise different types of abusive behaviours and therefore relate that to possible situations that they might find themselves in. Several of the adolescents spoke about this, but the following represents generally what was discussed:

> 1B: The abusive cycle . . . That was very clear on like how you'd be able to see in a relationship so you knew all the stages and would know what to do about it.

The theme, therefore, represents how the experiential learning was in effect transferred from the game and online interactions to interactions that might take place face-to-face. A second substantive theme concerned the experiential learning environment which reflected the factors and characteristics that were embedded within the game that then enable experiential learning to happen. The experiential learning environment comprised themes of familiar everyday technology, feedback and merging the cyber world into day-to-day reality.

Familiar everyday technology

The adolescents identified that the use of everyday technology was what was required for them to learn and therefore they saw the game in a positive light. This can be seen in three slightly different although closely linked ways. First, they liked the fact that learning about ADV was named and presented as an online *game* and not an intervention. It did seem that this format, i.e. a digital game, was the type of technology that the adolescents preferred, suggesting it would be more appealing to use and perhaps therefore encourage learning:

> 2A: It was good because most computer games are animated anyway and that's like what kids like to see so it would have appealed to them more.

Second, playing the game was also deemed to be a positive experience because it was completed electronically and doing activities on computers seemed to be recognised as the most appropriate and suitable way to receive and process data or information. That is to say using a computer for the adolescents appears to be the 'norm' and the preferred (or possibly expected) way to do things.

> 3A: It's better because erm, children are more like focused on the media now and it was good that it was like on computers because that's what kids focus on.

Finally, the fact that playing the game involved using familiar technologies was another factor that the adolescents identified as being positive and a strength of the learning environment that they had participated in:

> 3C: Probably the fact you had like all the different tools that you could use like you had the GPS, and like the texts and the emails and then, when it done the little videos as well like, instead of just explaining what happened . . .

Feedback

The adolescents identified that feedback was an important part of the learning environment. It has been suggested that with digital learning the system should provide students with encouraging feedback as this increases motivation, that this should be immediate as this helps the student to identify any problematic parts of their learning (Nokelainen 2006), and that it is an opportunity not just to take stock of the progress they have made, but also to improve their self-regulation (Corbalan et al. 2009). Feedback also enables individuals to acquire deep learning (Erhel and Jamet, 2013).

Feedback seems to be a feature of the learning environment that was seen as important and useful by those who played the game. In one conversation when discussing why feedback was good, it was decided that it:

2A: Made me understand it, there was lots of different scenarios, lots of options and things you could choose from and then about the abuse you saw, the different things to look at it clearly showed you what to look out for.

2D: Gave you a sense that if you did something good then it would tell you if you did it good, but if you did something bad it would tell you why it was bad not just oh you did it wrong . . . it was just helpful and it told us how we could do better.

Although some of the students thought that the feedback was repetitive in places, the value of the feedback was still acknowledged:

3A: It [feedback] was repetitive because we've heard of it before so it was like reinforcing it.

While feedback was seen as a positive aspect, it was also suggested how the feedback that was presented could be improved. It was suggested that it would be helpful to be given a final solution, and being told what the best options were in each circumstance would improve the feedback mechanism of the game:

1B: I think it would have been better if at the end it told you that this *is* definitely the best way to do it because it was just kind of you guessing so you could have been wrong and you wouldn't know which of the other ones is the right one.

Merging the cyber world into day-to-day reality

A really interesting factor that came out from the focus group was the extent to which adolescents felt immersed within the game world as they talked about what they were doing as being a reality. For example:

1A: You're in a classroom, you've got to talk to people, find stuff out.

1C: That you become a character then sort of go through their experiences I guess.

It seemed to be taking on the role of the characters, and importantly characters that were believable, that was particularly appealing to the adolescents. This fact made it like a reality for them.

1B: And you kind of got into it because you were almost like playing a character you kind of got into it more than if you were just kind of answering questions.

2B: They [the characters] were believable.

Making the situational factors realistic and in line with what the adolescents would in fact experience normally on a day-to-day basis meant that their cyber world was intrinsically linked to reality:

> 2E: It's like you're actually like playing as yourself, like going around a school when you're in a school yourself and it relates to what you are.

> 2A: They [the characters] were around our age and experiencing the same problems that we would.

A third major thematic area reflected the tension between online game education and traditional teaching. Using an online game as a form of education was seen as an effective learning experience and was compared with traditional teaching methods which were also seen to have a place in the adolescents' learning:

> 1A: I think people are more likely to listen more instead of just a teacher telling you stuff; people will actually interact with the game because it's just you and a computer.

However, what was debated was whether the game should be used for a whole lesson, or used as one component within a lesson. Some of the adolescents argued that the digital approach was appropriate for the whole lesson:

> 2D: It doesn't feel like you're on the computer for an hour because it's like a game but it's the whole lesson that you're going to need to actually play the game.

Others, however, noted that while they agreed that the game was a welcome addition, this should form part of a lesson, or be used in conjunction with other traditional teaching approaches:

> 1A: Possibly people, I don't know but people could feel like it's a bit detached, a bit like this is just a game it isn't going to happen so I think like it should be mixed with a few teacher-based lessons to like say this can happen, this is a real thing.

Opinion was divided on the role of the teacher. Teachers were identified as useful sources of information, and yet in contrast the presence of a teacher was perceived as reducing the openness with which young people may interact with the lesson content, which in turn may be counterproductive:

> 1B: But with a teacher you can like ask questions and say yeah I don't get that and stuff.

2A: And it's not like, it's quite private as well because you don't have to, whereas teachers encourage you to say stuff in front of everybody else but if it's just you, you're more likely to say something that you'd actually want to say.

Thoughts and observations for future developments

It was clear from our experience throughout the project that, consistent with previous studies, both teachers and young people welcomed the development of a digital resource that could be used to inform lessons concerning ADV. The focus groups in particular raised some interesting issues that need to be considered when designing such interventions.

First, the extent to which young people found the game immersive was surprising. The game graphics were very basic, not three-dimensional, and the game did not use a first-person perspective. Indeed, the artistry more closely reflected that of a graphic novel. What this means, however, is that care and attention needs to be paid to how characters and scenarios are represented. Designers need to carefully consider what kind of reality they should portray within game scenarios. For example, when designing the characters the project team had discussions regarding the diversity of characters in terms of apparent ethnicity and disability, and also in terms of how slim female characters should be drawn.

Second, it was clear that the actual format of the game was acceptable to students, although the extent to which lessons on ADV should rely on digital game content relative to traditional didactic content was less clear. What the focus groups did highlight, however, was that young people felt more at ease being open in their decision making in ADV scenarios when presented through a digital game, than they would have been in more traditional teacher-led discussions. This is consistent with emerging data indicating that character-driven online methods (chatbots) lead to greater disclosure of personal information than more traditional interview approaches (Crutzen et al. 2011). Consequently, it is likely that classroom-based interventions that combine the didactic presentation of 'factual' material by the teacher (which is valued by students as giving the issue validity) with more immersive scenario-based learning components delivered through digital media may be the most beneficial combination.

Third, it was clear that the technological capabilities of schools varied considerably, particularly in relation to the specification of computer hardware and software. Practical issues with game content being slow to load, and at times the synchronisation between video and audio channels being lost, impacted on the learning experience of the young people. Consequently, digital games need to be designed using software platforms that can be used on older hardware platforms in order to be of use to classroom-based teaching.

Finally, although teachers and schools welcomed the idea of a digital game for teaching on the issue of ADV, it was clear that the opportunities for using the game varied considerably from school to school. Moreover, the transient and responsive nature of some school curricula meant that when we thought we had a five-week implementation window, this could then be removed at the last minute as the head teacher had decided that the school would be using the identified implementation slot for something else. This perhaps reflects the fact that the identified implementation slot was that usually used for Personal Social and Health Education (PSHE), a non-compulsory component of the curriculum, which could therefore be treated as flexible in contrast to other components of the timetable that could not be. Clearly, if ADV education is going to form part of school curricula then it needs formal support and backing from both school teachers and governors as well as local authorities and government. It was clear to us that there is a genuine need for ADV to form part of the school curriculum. On the basis of piloting the game in one class of 25 children, two children approached their school counselling service as the game led them to question the health of their parents' relationship. Consequently, education concerning ADV can not only help young people deal with their own problematic relationships, but also lead them to safety away from the harm of other unhealthy relationships.

References

Abraham, C. and Michie, S. (2008) 'A taxonomy of behaviour change techniques used in interventions', *Health Psychology*, 27: 379–87.

Arnab, S., Brown, K., Clarke, S., Dunwell, I., Lim, T., Suttie, N. and de Freitas, S. (2013) 'The development approach of a pedagogically-driven serious game to support relationship and sex education (RSE) within a classroom setting', *Computers and Education*, 69: 15–30.

Barter, C., McCarry, M., Berridge, D. and Evans, K. (2009) *Partner Exploitation and Violence in Teenage Intimate Relationships*, London: NSPCC.

Bowen, E. and Walker, K. (2015) *The Psychology of Violence in Adolescent Romantic Relationships*, London: Palgrave.

Bowen, E., Holdsworth, E., Leen, E., Sorbring, E., Helsing, B., Jaans, S. and Awouters, V. (2013) 'Northern European adolescent attitudes toward dating violence', *Violence and Victims*, 28: 619–34.

Bowen, E., Walker, K., Mawer, M., Holdsworth, E., Sorbring, E., Helsing, B., Awouters, V. and Jans, S. (2014) '"It's like you're actually playing as yourself": development and preliminary evaluation of *Green Acres High*, a serious game-based primary intervention to combat adolescent dating violence', *Psychosocial Intervention*, 23: 43–55.

Charles, D. and McAlister, M. (2004) 'Integrating ideas about invisible playgrounds from play theory into online educational digital games', in M. Rauterberg (ed.) *Entertaining Computing: ICEC 2004*, Berlin and Heidelberg: Springer-Verlag.

Connolly, T.M., Boyle, E.A., MacArthur, E., Hainey, T. and Boyle, J.M. (2012) 'A systematic literature review of empirical evidence on computer games and serious games', *Computers and Education*, 59: 661–86.

Corbalan, G., Kester, L. and Van Merrienboer, J.J.G. (2009) 'Dynamic task selection: effects of feedback and learner control on efficiency and motivation', *Learning and Instruction*, 19: 455–65.

Council of Europe (2011) *Convention on Preventing and Combating Violence against Women and Domestic Violence*, Brussels: Council of Europe.

Crutzen, R., Peters, G.J.Y., Portugal, S.D., Fisser, E.M. and Grolleman, J.J. (2011) 'An artificially intelligent chat agent that answers adolescents' questions related to sex, drugs, and alcohol: an exploratory study', *Journal of Adolescent Health*, 48: 514–19.

Dempsey, J.V., Haynes, L.L., Lucassen, B.A. and Casey, M.S. (2002) 'Forty simple computer games and what they could mean to educators', *Simulation and Gaming*, 33: 157–68.

Erhel, S. and Jamet, E. (2013) 'Digital game-based learning: impact of instructions and feedback on motivation and learning effectiveness', *Computers and Education*, 67: 156–67.

Exner-Cortens, D., Eckenrode, J. and Rothman, E. (2013) 'Longitudinal associations between teen dating violence victimization and adverse health outcomes', *Pediatrics*, 131: 71–8.

Family Violence Project (2007) *Save the Date: a curriculum for teens on developing healthy dating relationships*. Santa Ana, CA: Family Violence Project.

Gamberini, L., Marchetti, F., Martino, F. and Spagnolli, A. (2009) 'Designing a serious game for young users: the case of Happy Farm', *Annual Review of CyberTherapy and Telemedicine*, 7: 77–81.

Gilliam, M., Jagoda, P., Jaworski, E., Hebert, L.E., Lyman, P. and Wilson, M.C. (2016) '"Because if we don't talk about it, how are we going to prevent it?" Lucidity, a narrative-based digital game about sexual violence', *Sex Education*, 16: 391–404.

Hainey, T., Connolly, T.M., Stansfield, M. and Boyle, E.A. (2011) 'Evaluation of a game to teach requirements collection and analysis in software engineering at tertiary education level', *Computers and Education*, 56: 21–35.

Hoffmann, L. (2009) 'Learning through games', *Communications of the ACM*, 52: 21–2.

Home Office and Women's Aid (n.d.) *Expect Respect: a toolkit for addressing teenage relationship abuse in key stages 3, 4 and 5*. Online. Available at www.gov.uk/government/uploads/system/uploads/attachment_data/file/97773/teen-abusetoolkit.pdf (accessed 28 February 2017).

Johnson, W.L., Giordano, P.C., Manning, W.D. and Longmore, M.A. (2015) 'The age–IPV curve: changes in the perpetration of intimate partner violence during adolescence and young adulthood', *Journal of Youth and Adolescence*, 44: 708–26.

Ke, F. (2013) 'Computer-game-based tutoring of mathematics', *Computers and Education*, 60: 448–57.

Kebritchi, M. and Hirumi, A. (2008) 'Examining the pedagogical foundations of modern educational computer games', *Computers and Education*, 51: 1729–43.

Kovačević, I., Minović, M., Milovanović, M., de Pablos, P.O. and Starčević D. (2013) 'Motivational aspects of different learning contexts: "My mom won't let me play this game . . .", *Computers in Human Behavior*, 29: 354–63.

Leen, E., Sorbring, E., Mawer, M., Holdsworth, E., Helsing, B. and Bowen, E. (2013) 'Prevalence, dynamic risk factors and the efficacy of primary interventions for adolescent dating violence: an international review', *Aggression and Violent Behavior*, 18: 159–74.

Majumdar, D., Koch, P., Lee, H., Contento, I., Islas, A. and Fu, D. (2012) '"Creature-101": using a virtual reality serious game to promote healthy eating and physical activity behaviors among middle school students', *Journal of Nutrition Education and Behavior*, 44: S38.

Mellecker, R.R., Witherspoon, L. and Watterson, T. (2013) 'Active learning: educational experiences enhanced through technology-driven active game play', *Journal of Educational Research*, 106: 352–9.

Men for Change (1994) *Healthy Relationships: a violence-prevention curriculum*, Nova Scotia: Men for Change.

Nokelainen, P. (2006) 'An empirical assessment of pedagogical usability criteria for digital learning material with elementary school students', *Journal of Educational Technology and Society*, 9: 178–97.

Rose, D.H., Meyer, A. and Hitchcock, C. (2005) *The Universally Designed Classroom: accessible curriculum and digital technologies*, Cambridge, MA: Harvard Education Press.

Sears, H.A., Byers, E.S., Whelan, J.J. and Saint-Pierre, M. (2006) '"If it hurts you, then it is not a joke": adolescents' ideas about girls' and boys' use and experience of abusive behavior in dating relationships', *Journal of Interpersonal Violence*, 21: 1191–207.

Shin, N., Sutherland, L.M., Norris, C.A. and Soloway, E. (2012) 'Effects of game technology on elementary student learning in mathematics', *British Journal of Educational Technology*, 43: 540–60.

Shorey, R.C., Fite, P.J., Choi, H., Cohen, J.R., Stuart, G.L. and Temple, J.R. (2015) 'Dating violence and substance use as longitudinal predictors of adolescents' risky sexual behavior', *Prevention Science*, 16: 853–61.

Smetana, L.K. and Bell, R.L. (2012) 'Computer simulations to support science instruction and learning: a critical review of the literature', *International Journal of Science Education*, 34: 1337–70.

Stonard, K.E., Bowen, E., Walker, K. and Price, S.A. (2015) '"They'll always find a way to get to you": technology use in adolescent romantic relationships and its role in dating violence and abuse', *Journal of Interpersonal Violence*. Doi: 10.1177/0886260515590787.

Sung, H.Y. and Hwang, G.J. (2013) 'A collaborative game-based learning approach to improving students' learning performance in science courses', *Computers and Education*, 63: 43–51.

Temple, J., Shorey, R., Fite, P., Stuart, G. and Le, V. (2013) 'Substance use as a longitudinal predictor of the perpetration of teen dating violence', *Journal of Youth and Adolescence*, 42: 596–606.

Thompson, D., Baranowski, T., Buday, R., Baranowski, J., Thompson, V., Jago, R. and Griffith, M.J. (2010) 'Serious video games for health: how behavioral science guided the development of a serious video game', *Simulation and Gaming*, 41: 587–606.

Virvou, M. and Katsionis, G. (2008) 'On the usability and likeability of virtual reality games for education: the case of VR-ENGAGE', *Computers and Education*, 50: 154–78.

Walsh, C. (2010) 'Systems-based literacy practices: digital games research, gameplay and design', *Australian Journal of Language and Literacy*, 33: 24–40.

Wolfe, D.A., Crooks, C., Jaffe, P., Chiodo, D., Hughes, R., Ellis, W. and Donner, A. (2009) 'A school-based program to prevent adolescent dating violence', *Archives of Pediatrics and Adolescent Medicine*, 163: 692–9.

5

VIOLENCE AND ABUSE IN YOUNG PEOPLE'S INTIMATE RELATIONSHIPS

Interface of gender, prevalence, impact and implications for prevention

Christine Barter

Introduction

This chapter outlines the issue of interpersonal violence and abuse (IPVA), including controlling behaviours, in the intimate relationships of young people aged 13 to 17 years old. Findings from three studies, undertaken by the author alongside colleagues, are used to demonstrate the prevalence and impact of IPVA in young relationships, including some exploration of young people's own narratives and understandings. Two of the studies (Barter et al. 2009; Wood et al. 2011) explored physical, sexual and emotional forms of IPVA in the UK. The third study, *Safeguarding Teenage Intimate Relationships*, known as '*STIR*' (Barter et al. 2015), addressed the ways in which new technologies were used in young people's relationships to reinforce other forms of face-to-face IPVA as well as constituting a discrete form of abuse. Building on these findings, the second half of the chapter addresses what we can do to prevent this form of abuse in young people's lives, and discusses the app that was developed as part of the *STIR* project.

Most international research on IPVA in young people's relationships has addressed three forms of abuse: physical, sexual and emotional/psychological. However, more recent studies have sought to explore the issue of abuse though new technologies, examining one or more of the following components: emotional online abuse (e.g. posting nasty/derogatory online messages); controlling behaviour (e.g. using mobile phones or social networking sites to try and control who someone can be friends with, where they go or how they dress); surveillance (e.g. constantly checking on what partners have been doing or who they have been seeing, demanding passwords to online social media accounts); social isolation (e.g. attempting to isolate partners from friends by posting untrue/derogatory messages from their phones, etc.); and coerced sexting. It is important to remember that in practice different forms of IPVA often intersect.

Research methodology

Two of the research studies used a mixed-method approach combining a school-based survey with in-depth semi-structured interviews with young people aged 14 to 17 years old. The first study (Barter et al. 2009) explored the use of emotional, physical and sexual forms of violence in adolescent relationships through a non-representative survey of 1,350 young people from 15 schools across England, Scotland and Wales and 91 interviews with young people. The second mixed-method project (Barter et al. 2015) also addressed the emerging issue of abuse through new technologies, including controlling behaviours and pressured sexting in Bulgaria, Cyprus, England, Italy and Norway. These countries were chosen to reflect differential levels of gender equality (Eurobarometer 2010) and use of new technology as reported in the EU kids online survey (Livingstone et al. 2011). The project included: expert workshops across the five countries; a non-representative survey (n=4,500) of young people from 45 schools; 100 interviews; and the development of an app for young people to explore their own relationship experiences, and to identify signs of risk and sources of support. The sampling framework ensured a balance by gender, schools from rural and urban areas and localities of economic diversity. Both studies facilitated young people's participation through youth advisory groups. The qualitative study (Wood et al. 2011) explored the IPVA experiences and views of more 'disadvantaged' young people (n=82) from a range of UK settings including young parent projects, young offender institutions, pupil referral units for excluded pupils, residential children's homes and foster care.

Findings

This section reports findings on prevalence rates and impact of IPVA victimisation in young people's relationships alongside young people's own narrative experiences and views. These are contextualised through comparison with two recent international meta-analyses on IPVA in young people's relationships.

In both surveys only young people who reported a partner, defined as someone they had been intimate with on a casual or long-term basis, were included in the IPVA analysis. This equated to 88 per cent (n=1185) for the 2009 survey and 72 per cent (n=3277), for the 2015 survey. All young people who reported a partner were asked how often they had experienced a specific abusive behaviour from a previous or current partner. Respondents could choose from never, once, a few times, often. In the following section all respondents who answered once or more have been combined into a single abuse category for analysis.

Emotional abuse/controlling behaviour

The 2009 study did not substantially differentiate between online and offline forms of emotional abuse and controlling behaviour, except in respect of one component (use of mobile phones/internet to humiliate/threaten). Overall, 75 per cent of girls and 50 per cent of boys reported some aspect of emotional abuse from a partner; this represented a significant gender difference. The most commonly reported behaviours were controlling behaviour and surveillance, although it was not known if these behaviours occurred online or offline:

> Like when I'd be out with my friends and he'd drag me off and say he didn't want me out any longer and I'd got to go in and it could be like half past six.
>
> *(female, Barter et al. 2009)*

Controlling behaviours were often normalised within young people's relationships. Wood et al. (2011) found that two-thirds of female participants compared with one-third of male participants reported some form of emotional violence, most often controlling behaviour through mobile phones. Around half of young women thought that control was an integral aspect of an intimate relationship and therefore normalised their partner's controlling behaviour. In contrast none of the boys reported this; most stated that their female partners' attempts at control were unacceptable. Few girls said they felt able to challenge the control they experienced, due to fear of negative repercussions:

> Mm. And then if I go out he'll just go mad and then just basically I'll just end up crying and go back home. So I'd just rather stay in . . . Which was a mistake really because then he used to do that all the time then, and then obviously he had something over me.
>
> *(female, Barter et al. 2009)*

Conversely, boys stated they either ignored the behaviour or would end the relationship if their partner's controlling behaviour continued:

Interviewer: How did you deal with it [constant phoning]?
Male respondent: I turned my phone off.

> *(Barter et al. 2009)*

Building on the above research, the 2015 survey separated face-to-face emotional abuse and abuse through new technologies. Across the five European countries, between 31 and 59 per cent of young women and 19 and 41 per cent of young men reported experiencing one or more of the four abusive behaviours from a partner, which is similar to the finding of Stonard et al. (2014) who reported that around half of all young people reported some form of emotional abuse from a partner. (See Table 5.1.)

Young men in England and Norway reported the lowest levels of face-to-face emotional violence. Only in England and Norway were significant gender differences found: girls were more likely to report emotional victimisation compared with boys.

TABLE 5.1 Percentage of respondents reporting types of IPVA by country and gender

Country	Gender	Emotional	Online	Physical	Sexual
Bulgaria	Female	41	47	11	21
	Male	35	43	15	25
Cyprus	Female	31	45	10	17
	Male	34	43	9	19
England	Female	48	48	22	41
	Male	27	25	12	14
Italy	Female	59	40	9	35
	Male	41	46	13	39
Norway	Female	32	38	18	28
	Male	19	20	8	9

Source: adapted from Barter et al. 2015: 27.

Online abuse

The online abuse measure used in the 2015 survey built on our previous interview findings and emergent online measures in the wider literature (Draucker and Martsolf 2010; Marganski and Fauth 2013; Zweig et al. 2013). The components sought to examine four main aspects of online abuse: emotional abuse; control; surveillance; and isolation from support. The overall rate for experiencing some form of online violence was around 40 per cent for both young women and young men in each country, which is slightly lower than reported elsewhere (Stonard et al. 2014; Wincentak et al. 2017). However, young men in England and Norway reported much lower levels of online abuse compared with young people in other countries (around 23 per cent), although the impact of online abuse could be just as devastating:

> of all the [Facebook and SMS] messages it was the message where she tried to convince me to commit suicide that was the hardest. She wrote that you don't dare it, you will never succeed . . . [after he attempted suicide she sent another, it said] 'I am sorry you were not successful.'
>
> *(male from Norway, Barter et al. 2015)*

Reflecting the 2009 survey findings, controlling behaviour and surveillance were the most commonly experienced forms of online violence for both young women and young men:

> He began to talk dirty to me, calling me nasty things, like 'go to the kitchen, whore', but I didn't do as he wanted, I am not a slave . . .[He posted an old picture saying that his girlfriend had been unfaithful to him with a girl] and then he kept writing these nasty comments, and people started commenting . . . really horrible stuff.
>
> *(female from Norway, Barter et al. 2015)*

This gender divide in respect of online victimisation, where pressured sexting and unwanted sharing of sexual images is primarily experienced by girls, has also been reported by others (Draucker and Martsolf 2010; Wood et al. 2015; Zweig et al. 2013). In our studies, some males openly regarded online forms of abuse as acceptable or even appropriate:

> To have your girlfriend 'like' photos of people she doesn't know isn't such a nice thing to see in Facebook ... when she does that it's as if she is saying she doesn't want me ... I don't want another man to come anywhere near her ... I tell her not to wear certain clothes ...
>
> *(male from Cyprus, Barter et al. 2015)*

Sexual violence

The same measure of sexual violence, which incorporated both pressure and physical force, was used in the 2009 and 2015 surveys. Overall, 35 per cent of girls and 16 per cent of boys reported sexual victimisation in the 2009 survey, most often pressure. As with emotional abuse this represented a significant gender difference:

> See with my relationship it wasn't up to me (when to have sex). But when it happens it just kind of happens and then afterwards you think oh my god.
>
> *(female, Barter et al. 2009)*

Rates of sexual violence across the European countries ranged from 17 to 41 per cent for young women and 9 to 25 per cent for young men. Again, most young people reported coercive sexual pressure rather than physical force. The 2015 survey also showed that the majority of young people reported this coercion occurred face-to-face or both face-to-face and online; very few reported online pressure in isolation. Young women in England and Norway reported the highest rates, with one in three reporting some form of unwanted sexual activity:

> I thought we were going to somewhere else and he led me to a park and started like pushing me around and forcing me to do things I didn't want to do and, and he pushed my head down so hard. I was sick everywhere and then they just left me.
>
> *(female from England, Barter et al. 2015)*

Wood et al. (2011) found that half of the girls in the qualitative study of disadvantaged young people in England reported experiences of sexual violence. A quarter stated this involved physical force. Only a small minority of boys reported sexual violence. Many girls did not recognise, or normalised, the seriousness of their experiences of sexual violence and were therefore less likely to seek help, reflecting the interview findings from the mixed-method studies. Many girls across studies and countries reported feeling uncertain about what they wanted sexually from their relationship or what was 'expected' of them:

Interviewer: So were you ever forced into having sex?
Female respondent: Yeah, quite a few times . . . it's quite horrible, I was only young, well I wasn't really really young, I wasn't . . . like when I was 12, it was like when I was 13.

(female, Wood et al. 2011)

Physical violence

As with sexual violence the same measure of physical victimisation was used across both surveys. The 2009 survey found that 25 per cent of girls and 18 per cent of boys reported physical victimisation, a significant gender difference:

> I only went out with him for a week. And then . . . 'cos I didn't want to do what he wanted to (have sexual intercourse) he just started . . . picking on me and hitting me.
>
> *(female, Barter et al. 2009)*

The 2015 survey identified that between 9 and 22 per cent of young women and 8 to 15 per cent of young men across the five countries reported some form of physical violence:

> The boy should be the boss. The girl should do everything that he asks. But he should treat her well . . . I said to her: Let's go to dance! I was a bit drunk. She did not want to. I took her out and started beating her.
>
> *(male from Bulgaria, Barter et al. 2015)*

Almost one in five young women in England and Norway reported having experienced physical violence compared with one in 10 in other countries. Some young women even suggested this was deserved:

> And he raised his fist to hit me . . . and I was thinking . . . I know it sounds stupid but . . . I felt as if I deserved it, but I was scared.
>
> *(female, Barter et al. 2009)*

As European research on adult domestic violence (DV) has shown, the willingness of participants to report their experiences is often heavily influenced by how DV is viewed in different countries (FRA 2014). Countries with higher gender equality and greater DV awareness also often report the highest levels of DV. This may be because in these countries DV is viewed as a social and political rather than a personal and therefore private problem. The *STIR* expert meetings (Barter et al. 2015) and the young people's advisory groups identified that England and Norway had the highest levels of awareness in respect of interpersonal abuse in young people's relationships, and young women from these two countries reported the highest levels of physical and sexual violence in the 2015 survey. It may therefore be that female respondents from the other countries were more likely to under-report their experiences of physical and sexual violence, rather than that the actual prevalence of IVPA was less than in England and Norway.

The 2015 survey findings are consistent with the two recent data syntheses (Stonard et al. 2014; Wincentak et al. 2017) which found that approximately 20 per cent of young people experience some form of physical violence from a partner, irrespective of gender, but previous studies suggest adolescent females report more severe forms of IPVA (Barter et al. 2009; Foshee 1996; Wolitzky-Taylor et al. 2008).

The impact of IPVA

Once impact is considered alongside prevalence, the gendered nature of IPVA becomes more salient. Our survey findings showed that girls more frequently report a negative subjective impact to their victimisation compared with boys (Barter et al. 2009, 2015). Most commonly girls report feeling scared, humiliated and upset, whilst boys who reported a negative consequence most often report feeling angry or annoyed (Barter et al. 2009, 2015; Wood et al. 2011). Jackson et al. (2000) in their New Zealand study also reported that girls experienced more negative emotional responses to IPVA victimisation than did boys. Other studies show that girls are more likely to be hurt or require medical attention than boys, whilst boys report laughing about the violence perpetrated against them (Foshee 1996; Molidor et al. 2000).

Far fewer young people reported a negative consequence in relation to emotional and, to a lesser degree, online forms of abuse. Only 31 per cent of girls and 6 per cent of boys reported a negative impact to emotional victimisation in the 2009 survey, although this did significantly increase when a behaviour or behaviours were reported to occur frequently. Looking at data on online abuse from the 2015 survey, between 49 and 83 per cent of young women and 28 and 41 per cent of young men reported a negative impact. As with emotional violence these proportions increased if the behaviour occurred frequently or if more than one form of online abuse was used. This illustrates that it is the overall patterning of emotional and online forms of abuse which causes the most distress rather than an isolated incidence, as was more the case for physical and sexual forms of violence, especially for girls.

Previous research has also identified that a range of adverse health outcomes are associated with IPVA victimisation in adolescence, including suicidal behaviours, mental health problems, depression, eating disorders, substance and alcohol use, pregnancy outcomes and physical injuries (Exner-Cortens et al. 2013; Silverman et al. 2001; van Dulmen et al. 2012). A recent review by the current author and a colleague identified that evidence indicates that IPVA health impacts appear to be more severe for girls than boys (Barter and Stanley 2016). Adolescent IPVA is also one of the strongest precursors for female IPVA victimisation in adulthood (Exner-Cortens et al. 2013, van Dulmen et al. 2012).

Our findings, alongside international research, clearly show that IPVA in young people's relationships represents a major social issue and public health concern. Having outlined the scale and impact of the problem we now turn to explore the evidence on effective IPVA prevention programmes for young people and discuss the development of the app within the *STIR* project.

Prevention programmes

Although robust evaluations of IPVA prevention programmes with adolescents are increasing (Wolfe et al. 2009), globally there remains a substantial shortage of robust evidence on their effectiveness. Many of the evaluated prevention programmes are from North America and it remains unclear how cultural differences, including differences in dating practices and gender norms, impact on implementation in other international contexts. Interventions are likely to be culturally specific and thus it is necessary to evaluate and adjust the intervention to fit the national or local context. One evidenced US programme was found to be ineffective within a European context (Hamby et al. 2012).

Three recent reviews provide us with a clear message regarding effective prevention programmes. A Cochrane systematic review (Fellmeth et al. 2013) found that programmes predominantly addressed IPVA attitudinal change, skills and knowledge transfer rather than measuring behavioural change. In conclusion, the review found no evidence that interventions were effective in reducing IPVA, although they did evidence changes in attitudes and knowledge. A slightly more recent meta-analysis by De La Rue et al. (2014) produced more promising results, with two randomised controlled trials (RCTs), *Safe Dates* (Foshee et al. 1998) and *Shifting Boundaries* (Taylor et al. 2013), showing long-term behavioural change (both were excluded from the Fellmeth et al. (2013) review owing to incomplete reporting and later publication respectively). In a review of peer sexual violence prevention *Safe Dates* and *Shifting Boundaries* were identified as the only effective interventions (DeGue et al. 2014).

Fellmeth et al. (2013) identified that less effective interventions tended to be short-term in duration, and lacked a clear structure and model of change. They recommend that further research evaluations on multi-component interventions, which include a whole-school approach, are a priority. The De La Rue et al. (2014) review recommended that future interventions more explicitly address skills and the role of peer norms in preventing IPVA.

A recent project (Stanley et al. 2015) systematically reviewed IPVA interventions for children and young people and held consultations with experts and young people. The authors report that three RCTs showed evidence of long-term behavioural change, the *Fourth R* programme (Wolfe et al. 2009) being judged to be particularly robust. From this they provide a number of key messages, including:

- effective programmes challenge social norms including stereotypical gender norms, power differentials and victim-blaming attitudes, and harness pro-social peer pressure to change attitudes;
- both young people and experts argued for the value of drama/theatre and narrative;
- authenticity was achieved through material that delivered emotional charge and made '*it real*' and enhanced when delivered by experts or young people themselves;
- whole population interventions harness peer group power but can also identify those at risk who require additional services;
- interventions must acknowledge diversity amongst children and young people;
- messages should be positively framed and avoid blame;
- values and attitudes of the peer group are crucial mechanisms for change;
- children's and young people's perceptions and experiences should be incorporated into interventions; and media and social media awareness campaigns can be a useful tool for engagement.

Common to all three reviews was the need to ensure prevention is based on a solid theory of change and that we are realistic about what different forms of prevention can achieve for different groups. Three main theories of change used in prevention programmes are: social cognitive theory; the social norms approach; and the theory of gender and power.

Social cognitive theory

Social cognitive theory, developed by Bandura (1986), has been widely used in public health interventions, including those addressing IPVA in adolescent relationships (for example Wolfe et al. 2009). Social cognitive theory holds that knowledge acquisition and attitudinal and behavioural change can be acquired through observing others within the context of social interactions, direct experiences and modelling positive responses. Observing a modelled behaviour can also prompt the viewer to re-evaluate current negative behaviour by replicating the observed behaviour.

One way of enabling this modelling and for this to feel authentic is through the use of drama. Stanley et al. (2015) found that young people themselves valued interventions that made learning 'real' for them and that deliver emotional 'charge'. Both the *Safe Dates* and the *Fourth R* programmes incorporate aspects of drama which enables young people, through scene enactments, to both observe behaviour and practise conflict resolution skills (Joronen et al. 2008; Wolfe et al. 2009). Involving young people themselves in the creation and delivery of such messages increased their authenticity for a young audience (Joronen et al. 2008).

Social norms approach

A wide range of IPVA prevention programmes are underpinned by a social norms approach (Stanley et al. 2015) that seeks to challenge behaviours that reinforce violence as a social norm. A strong evidence base has been developed by bodies such as the World Health Organization (WHO 2009) to support the use of interventions that challenge norms, assumptions and behaviour that tolerate violence. Healthy relationship norms, supported by wider school learning through teacher training, are promoted to replace anti-social norms.

The theory of gender and power

A very large literature, grounded in feminism or sociology of gender, recognises the social and institutional mechanisms that constrain women's and girls' daily practices through gender-based inequities and gendered expectations (Connell 1987). Empirical evidence has shown that negative gendered attitudes are significantly connected to both experiencing and perpetrating IPVA in adolescent relationships (Barter et al. 2015). The gender and power theoretical model hypothesises that exposure to traditional beliefs around gendered cultural norms associated with hegemonic masculinity (active, controlling) and femininity (passive, vulnerable) serves to reinforce IPVA norms and behaviour.

A growing tendency for interventions to target young men with negative and blaming discourses (Stanley et al. 2015) leads to defensive reactions and disengagement (Donovan et al. 2008). To avoid this, the blaming or risk approach should be avoided and the emphasis should be placed on positive messages around masculinity (Stanley et al. 2015), which challenge constraining gender norms and uphold a gender-transformative approach (WHO 2009). Conversely, programmes that uphold traditional and stereotypical conceptions of masculinity can further reinforce harmful gender norms (Fleming et al. 2014).

App development

Within the *STIR* project, each country convened a young people's advisory group (YPAG) consisting of between 10 and 15 members aged 14 to 17, who worked alongside the research teams for the duration of the project. One of the main priorities of the YPAGs across the five countries was to work with the researchers and wider experts to determine the aims of the app and how best to operationalise these, ensuring their relevance and appropriateness across the five country contexts. To aid communication across the YPAGs an online interactive discussion forum was set up where groups took turns to set a specific question or discussion point related to the project which all five groups debated. The country-specific discussions were then posted on the online board and these posts were then commented on, debated or elaborated on by the whole forum. All discussions were translated. This process enabled issues around IPVA definitions, terminology, cultural contents and peer norms to be explored.

For example, regarding terminology all young people felt that the term 'dating violence', widely adopted in US programmes, was not applicable within a European context. Instead they preferred the term 'relationship violence' which they felt reflected a wider range of relationship types: casual, short-term or longer-term. It was also felt to be important that the app resource did not presume heteronormativity so the generic term 'partner' was used to ensure inclusion. Building on this it was agreed that the app should highlight different forms of relationship, for example in the interactive story a variety of relationships were involved, including a same-sex relationship.

It was also clear from the online discussions that country-specific awareness around different aspects of IPVA existed and that certain forms of abuse, especially aspects of controlling behaviour and surveillance, were viewed with varying degrees of acceptance in some country contexts. The online forum provided a space where young people could debate these issues and challenge each other's assumptions in ways which did not produce a defensive response but enabled participants to have space to reflect on their understandings and challenge attitudes which reinforce IPVA. For example, in one discussion jealousy was presented as an acceptable reason to justify certain forms of controlling behaviour and online surveillance. Others questioned the validity of this and instead presented ways in which trust could be better developed within relationships to reduce feelings of insecurity.

This is not to say that a consensus was always achieved across groups or within groups; however, these dynamic online discussions provided a rich and culturally sensitive resource to support the app development. It was interesting that generally the commonalities across the groups were greater than the differences. All groups, for example, agreed that we should avoid using emotive terms such as victim, perpetrator, abuse and/or violence within the interactive aspects of the app as young people may become distressed if they felt these labels were being applied to them or their relationships. Instead an emphasis was placed on the benefits of a respectful relationship whilst unhealthy aspects were referred to as 'concerning' to reduce the chance of a defensive response.

The YPAGs wanted the app to be interactive but also felt that the format should be kept simple so that it did not look outdated quickly owing to rapid advances in technology. It was also felt that photographic images might appear country-specific so it was decided to restrict the format to text and graphics. The YPAGs agreed that the best way to raise young people's awareness of IPVA was through a quiz format. Two quizzes were developed: one addressed how a young person's partner behaved towards them and the other explored the young person's own relationship behaviour and attitudes. All questions were developed by young people together with the researchers. After each question the app user is asked how frequently this has occurred: never, sometimes or often. The user is then directed to a response depending on their answer – all responses were taken from the interactive message board or from the interviews with young people and seek to reinforce positive messages regarding respectful relationships as well as highlighting possible 'concerns'. For example, the aim of the 'Is your relationship rocking?' quiz was to identify issues around relationship victimisation. The 12 quiz questions were designed to help the user recognise 'the tricky situations that can arise in a relationship' through highlighting unhealthy components. If upon completion of the quiz a high number of risk factors are identified, the user is directed to a further section where advice on possible sources of support and help are provided. However, and as stated earlier, it was felt important that a young person should not be defined as an 'abuse victim' owing to the distress this may cause and instead responses highlighted their partner's concerning behaviour.

Similarly, the quiz to assess the young person's own relationship behaviour asks 'How great a partner are you?' The challenges to successfully engaging boys in IPVA prevention and awareness have already been addressed (Stanley et al. 2015). Interestingly, many male YPAG members stated that male users would be more likely to access the quiz if they felt it would help them get a partner! It was decided this might not be appropriate but that helping young people to think about how to get better at being in a relationship was acceptable.

An interactive story was also developed where the user determines how a number of relationships develop in different healthy and unhealthy ways. This resource enables young people who have not been in a relationship to explore the possible risks and contexts in which IPVA can occur as well as protective strategies. The app also provides sources of assistance and support in each country. Safety was paramount so an escape button was included to ensure the user could quickly leave the app if necessary. The prototype app was piloted with more than 120 young people across the five countries and received very positive feedback. The team are currently working towards undertaking a more in-depth evaluation of the app which is available from http://stiritapp.eu.

Conclusions

In conclusion it is clear from our research findings, alongside international evidence, that IPVA in young people's relationships represents a major concern, and that girls and young women experience the severest forms of IPVA and identify the most negative impacts. This form of violence, in all its connotations, requires a considered and comprehensive response. We know what effective prevention interventions look like but need to develop these, alongside children and young people, to reach beyond the North American contexts in which they have been evidenced. In the UK colleagues and I are beginning this process by transferring the *Safe Dates* and *Shifting Boundaries* interventions to the UK and undertaking RCTs to evaluate their effectiveness. However, public health prevention can only do so much and even effective interventions have been shown to have modest results. There is therefore a pressing need to ensure that, alongside prevention, direct and easily accessible services for young IPVA victims are developed that take their experiences seriously and work to ensure they are kept safe, and that abusive partners receive appropriate programmes and, where necessary, criminal justice responses.

References

Bandura, A. (1986) *Social Foundations of Thought and Action: a social cognitive theory*, Englewood Cliffs, NJ: Prentice-Hall.

Barter, C. and Stanley, N. (2016) 'Interpersonal violence and abuse in adolescent intimate relationships: mental health impact and implications for practice', *International Review of Psychiatry*, 28: 485–503.

Barter, C., McCarry, M., Berridge, D. and Evans, K. (2009) *Partner Exploitation and Violence in Teenage Intimate Relationships*, London: NSPCC.

Barter, C., Stanley, N., Wood, M., Aghtaie, N., Larkins, C., Øverlien, C., Lesta, S. and De Luca, N. (2015) *Safeguarding Teenage Intimate Relationships (STIR): connecting online and offline contexts and risks*. Online. Available at http://stiritup.eu/wp-content/uploads/2015/06/STIR-Exec-Summary-English.pdf (accessed 11 November 2016).

Connell, R.W. (1987) *Gender and Power: society, the person and sexual politics*, Cambridge: Polity Press.

De La Rue, L., Polanin, J., Espelage, D. and Pigott, T. (2014) 'School-based interventions to reduce dating and sexual violence: a systematic review', *Campbell Systematic Reviews*, 10(7). Online. Available at www.campbellcollaboration.org/lib/project/268/ (accessed 11 November 2016).

DeGue, S., Valle, L., Holy, M., Massetti, G., Matjasko, J. and Tharp, A. (2014) 'A systematic review of primary prevention strategies for sexual violence perpetration', *Aggression and Violent Behavior*, 19: 346–62.

Donovan, R.J., Jalleh, G., Fielder, L. and Ouschan R. (2008) 'When confrontational images may be counterproductive: reinforcing the case for pre-testing communications in sensitive areas', *Health Promotion Journal of Australia*, 19: 132–6.

Draucker, C.B. and Martsolf, D.S. (2010) 'The role of electronic communication technology in adolescent dating violence', *Journal of Child and Adolescent Psychiatric Nursing*, 23: 133–42.

Eurobarometer (2010) *Domestic Violence against Women Report*, Brussels: European Commission. Online. Available at http://ec.europa.eu/public_opinion/archives/ebs/ebs_344_en.pdf (accessed 11 November 2016).

Exner-Cortens, D., Eckenrode, J. and Rothman, E. (2013) 'Longitudinal associations between teen dating violence victimization and adverse health outcomes', *Pediatrics*, 131(1): 71–8.

Fellmeth, G.L., Heffernan, C., Nurse, J., Habibula, S. and Sethi, D. (2013) 'Educational and skills-based interventions for preventing relationship and dating violence in adolescents and young adults', *Cochrane Database Systematic of Reviews*, June 19(6): CD004534. Online. Available at http://onlinelibrary.wiley.com/doi/10.1002/14651858.CD004534.pub3/full (accessed 11 November 2016).

Fleming, P.J., Lee, J.G.L. and Dworkin, S.L. (2014) '"Real Men Don't": constructions of masculinity and inadvertent harm in public health interventions', *American Journal of Public Health*, 104: 1029–35.

Foshee, V. (1996) 'Gender differences in adolescent dating abuse prevalence, types, and injuries', *Health Education Research*, 11: 275–86.

Foshee, V.A., Bauman, K.E., Arriaga, X.B., Helms, R.W., Koch, G.G. and Linder, G.F. (1998) 'An evaluation of *Safe Dates*, an adolescent dating violence prevention program', *American Journal of Public Health*, 88: 45–50.

FRA (European Union Agency for Fundamental Rights) (2014) *Violence against Women: an EU-wide survey*. Online. Available at http://fra.europa.eu/sites/default/files/fra-2014-vaw-survey-main-results_en.pdf (accessed 11 November 2016).

Hamby, S., Nix, K., De Puy, J. and Monnier, S. (2012) 'Adapting dating violence prevention to francophone Switzerland: a story of intra-western cultural differences', *Violence and Victims*, 27: 33–42.

Jackson, S.M., Cram, F. and Seymour, F.W. (2000) 'Violence and sexual coercion in high school students' dating relationships', *Journal of Family Violence*, 15: 23–36.

Joronen, K.K., Rankin, S.H. and Åstedt-Kurki, P. (2008) 'School-based drama interventions in health promotion for children and adolescents: systematic review', *Journal of Advanced Nursing*, 63: 116–31.

Livingstone, S., Haddon, L., Görzig, A. and Ólafsson, K. (2011) *Risks and Safety on the Internet: the perspective of European children. Full findings and policy implications from the EU kids online survey of 9–16 year olds and their parents in 25 countries*, London: EU Kids Online Network. Online. Available at www.lse.ac.uk/media@lse/research/EUKidsOnline/EU%20 Kids%20II%20(2009-11)/EUKidsOnlineIIReports/D4FullFindings.pdf (accessed 11 November 2016).

Marganski, A. and Fauth, K. (2013) 'Socially interactive technology and contemporary dating: cross-cultural exploration of deviant behaviour among young adults in the modern, evolving technological world', *International Criminal Justice Review*, 23: 357–77.

Molidor, C., Tolman, R.M. and Kober, J. (2000) 'Gender and contextual factors in adolescent dating violence', *Prevention Researcher*, 7: 1–4.

Silverman, J.G., Raj, A., Mucci, L.A. and Hathaway, J.E. (2001) 'Dating violence against adolescent girls and associated substance use, unhealthy weight control, sexual risk behavior, pregnancy, and suicidality', *Journal of the American Medical Association*, 286: 572–9.

Stanley. N., Ellis, J., Farrelly, N., Hollinghurst, S. and Downe, S. (2015) 'Preventing domestic abuse for children and young people: a review of school-based interventions', *Children and Youth Services Review*, 59: 120–31.

Stonard, K., Bowen, E., Lawrence, T. and Price, S.A. (2014) 'The relevance of technology to the nature, prevalence and impact of adolescent dating violence and abuse: a research synthesis', *Aggression and Violent Behavior*, 19: 390–417.

Taylor, B.G., Stein, N., Mumford, E. and Woods, D. (2013) '*Shifting Boundaries*: an experimental evaluation of a dating violence prevention program in middle schools', *Prevention Science*, 14: 64–76.

van Dulmen, M.H.M., Klipfel, K.M., Mata, M.D, Schinka, K.C., Claxton, S.E., Swahn, M.H. and Bossarte, R.M. (2012) 'Cross-lagged effects between intimate partner violence victimization and suicidality from adolescence into adulthood', *Journal of Adolescent Health*, 51: 510–16.

Wincentak, K., Connolly, J. and Card, N. (2017) 'Teen dating violence: a meta-analytic review of prevalence rates', *Psychology of Violence,* 7: 224–41.

Wolfe, D.A., Crooks, C.V., Jaffe, P.G., Chiodo, D., Hughes, R., Ellis, W., Stitt, L. and Donner, A. (2009) 'A school-based program to prevent adolescent dating violence: a cluster randomized trial', *Archives of Pediatrics and Adolescent Medicine*, 163: 692–9.

Wolitzky-Taylor, K.B., Ruggiero, K.J., Danielson, C.K., Resnick, H.S., Hanson, R.F., Smith, D.W. and Kilpatrick, D.G. (2008) 'Prevalence and correlates of dating violence in a national sample of adolescents', *Journal of the American Academy of Child and Adolescent Psychiatry*, 47: 755–62.

Wood, M., Barter, C. and Berridge, D. (2011) *Standing On My Own Two Feet: disadvantaged young people and partner violence*, London: NSPCC.

Wood, M., Barter, C., Stanley, N., Aghtaie, N. and Larkins, C. (2015) 'Images across Europe: the sending and receiving of sexual images (sexting) and associations with intimate partner violence in young people's relationships', *Youth Services Review*, 59: 149–60.

WHO (2009) *Changing Cultural and Social Norms that Support Violence*, Geneva: World Health Organization. Online. Available at www.who.int/violence_injury_prevention/violence/norms.pdf (accessed 11 November 2016).

Zweig, J.M., Dank, M., Yahner, J. and Lachman, P. (2013) 'The rate of cyber dating abuse among teens and how it relates to other forms of teen dating violence', *Journal of Youth and Adolescence*, 42: 1063–77.

6

CAMPUS SAFETY PROJECT

Strategies, recommendations and obstacles in addressing gender-based violence on campuses

Clara Porter and Cathy Plourde

Introduction

American universities and colleges have long been expected to actively prevent, intervene and respond to gender-based violence (GBV) on campus. However, although Title IX, a federal law that prohibits discrimination on the basis of sex in any federally funded education programme or activity, was enacted in 1972, it has rarely been applied to GBV (USDOJ 2015). The US Department of Justice Office on Violence Against Women (OVW) was created in 1995 to administer the 1994 Violence against Women Act (VAWA) (USC 1994) and provides funding to universities to address GBV. The 2011 US Department of Education 'Dear Colleague' letter put universities nationwide on notice that GBV is covered under Title IX, gave a basic framework for response and prevention, and warned that federal financial aid dollars could be lost for noncompliance (USDOE OCR 2011). While much work remains, recent innovations hold real promise for change on and off campuses.

This chapter examines the inauguration of the *Campus Safety Project* (*CSP*) at the University of Southern Maine (USM) in 2010–13. It represents an overview of GBV prevention, education and response measures at one US university and provides recommendations in light of critical issues facing US campuses.

The start of the University of Southern Maine's *Campus Safety Project*

The OVW Campus Grant programme awarded USM three years of funding to design and implement a comprehensive response to GBV including policies and response protocols, training, prevention education and support for students. While the advocacy and tenacity of a small group of faculty and staff had succeeded in securing OVW funding for USM, the administration did not view GBV as a concern demanding dramatic action. Efforts to address GBV through awareness activities and academic efforts prior to 2010 were small-scale and staff training, risk reduction and response efforts occurred primarily within the Department of Residential Life. Prior to 2010, GBV incidents reported under the *Jeanne Clery Act* (Ward and Mann 2011) were implausibly low for a school of 9,000 students (no more than three per year) and Conduct Board cases had been overwhelmingly resolved in favour of students accused of GBV.

Clara Porter was hired as *CSP* Coordinator in March of 2010 and developed a programme based on the social-ecological model (Krug et al. 2002). This recognises the interplay of individual, relational, community and societal factors and uses an asset-based approach to change (Kretzmann and McKnight 1993), which seeks to identify and develop the skills, resources and ideas of a community working towards change. Porter's status as an outsider well acquainted with local service providers was useful in building trust on campus and crafting critical campus/community partnerships. Grant signatories represented academic and student services departments, campus police and conduct offices; community-based domestic violence and sexual assault (DV/SA) agencies; legal services programmes; and law enforcement. Representatives from each formed a Coordinating Committee (CC) to guide the project.

Response protocol

Historically, response to disclosures of GBV depended largely upon who the initial report was made to, with no consistency across USM's three campuses. The CC decided that revising the response protocols prior to the launch of major student awareness efforts would form the cornerstone to efficient, consistent response, key components of a strong safety net.

As the new protocol was crafted, the DV/SA agencies advocated for limiting the number of people involved once a student disclosed GBV, based on accepted best practice of limiting the number of times trauma survivors are compelled to retell their story (Woods 2000) and concern for student privacy. Conversely, Residential Life staff asserted that the more staff involved the greater the support. While these positions appear opposite, each desired to provide a 'victim-centred' response. Expert advice was sought and the CC agreed to shift control over response to the Title IX Coordinator or their designated deputy, thus limiting the number of people informed at the time of a disclosure.

In order to encourage reporting, provide support for survivors and ensure fair treatment of accused students, protocols and policies must protect the privacy of all involved. The *Respond, Refer, Report* protocol was developed as a clear and concise document which defined the role of university employees in responding to students disclosing GBV. It distinguished between confidentiality and privacy, ensuring that only the employee and the Title IX Coordinator would be aware of the disclosure until the student decided upon additional steps, if any. In the event of a perceived threat to the community, the student was to be kept informed of every step taken. Disclosure to mental health counsellors or ordained chaplains would remain confidential unless action was mandated as a result of a clear threat to self or others (USM 2016).

A confidential case review process was conducted by the Title IX Coordinator, advocates from DV/SA partner agencies, legal services representative (as relevant), campus police, *CSP* and other student life staff. The team met periodically to examine recent cases, tracing a path from disclosure to employee response, linkage with resources and final disposition. Case review revealed areas for adjustment and better coordination such as timeliness of response to a complaint, the location of conduct hearings, and the provision of intermediate supports for survivors such as housing and course changes.

Over the course of the grant, CC members had the opportunity to attend national conferences to increase their knowledge of GBV and best practices for prevention and intervention. The CC also attended a half-day training session, which aimed to:

- increase appreciation of the complexities of GBV;
- foster trust and relationships amongst CC members; and
- deepen commitment to change in the university response system.

The training session, based on the work of Lisak and Miller (2002), reviewed GBV perpetration and explored how common trauma responses such as partial memory, confusion and flat affect could appear to the untrained person as signs of deception. This training proved profound, especially for members of the Conduct Board as they recalled a recent case in which they had found against a complainant (victim) in part due to these same trauma behaviours.

Conduct code and policy revision

With the response protocol in place, the CC next turned to policies related to GBV and the Student Code of Conduct, which applied across the state's seven-campus university system. Conduct Office staff attended trainings and OVW-mandated conferences and compared University of Maine policies with those of other universities and against the current understanding of Title IX. Revision of the Code is undertaken by a statewide committee on a three-year schedule and instituting changes would have meant waiting two years. The Conduct Office ingeniously circumvented this restriction by starting with changes to internal protocols, dramatically improving USM response to cases of GBV far in advance of the approval of the revised Code and university policy.

Training

The CC recognised the need to establish a shared base of knowledge and practice campus-wide. Employees whose roles and level of student contact predicted student disclosures of GBV were first to be trained.

- Residential Life staff were trained to use de-escalation and grounding, to avoid asking questions about the incident, to encourage the student to contact a confidential community-based advocate, and to enlist the residential director who would engage the reporting protocol.
- *CSP* and DV/SA partners trained health and counselling staff on the signs of GBV in students seeking services, the prevalence of such crimes and the role of the community-based advocates. In year two, University Counseling instituted a daily 'on-call' counsellor to respond to crises including students coming through the *Respond, Refer, Report* protocol.
- The Conduct Office instituted an annual training on university protocols, reporting requirements and sanctions for the Conduct Board (comprising students, staff and faculty), including information on dynamics present in GBV, common perpetrator tactics and trauma-related behaviour.
- Training for campus police was conducted by community-based partners or was accessed online. Over time *CSP* succeeded in making training mandatory for all officers, increasing the baseline knowledge of many, but consistency in approach and sensitivity to various classes of students was not achieved.

A second tier of training included financial aid, academic counselling, administrative assistants and support staff, and departments employing large numbers of students, such as mail and dining services. Employees working in Financial Aid are uniquely positioned to assist students experiencing GBV as abusive partners may seek to impede financial aid awards as a way to exert control. Further, aid can be jeopardised if grades fall, which often occurs in the aftermath of GBV. Training prepared staff to recognise GBV and utilise the protocol effectively.

Foundational elements

CSP's educational programming was built upon four specific foundational assumptions: survivors are in the room, always; engagement of men must be multi-faceted; programming must meet the needs of diverse populations; and, community partner involvement is critical.

Survivors in the room

All *CSP* programmes acknowledged the fact of survivors being present amongst the participants. According to the US Department of Justice, 29 per cent of sexual assault and rape victims of all genders were under the age of 17 at the time of their assault (Greenfeld 1997) and a 2015 survey by Rutgers University revealed 24 per cent of undergraduate women report experiencing sexual assault prior to college (McMahon et al. 2015). Disclosures by participants of past or current experiences of GBV were frequent, particularly amongst staff and students receiving such training for the first time. All training included tools for self-care, provided linkage to resources, and included the presence of DV/SA advocates allowing for immediate support.

Engaging men

Men have a clear role to play in GBV prevention, interruption and response. *CSP*'s efforts to reach male students were sensitive to the stereotypical 'profiling' of fraternities and athletes; to men's generalised defensiveness on the subject of sexual assault; and to the misconception that men are perpetrators rather than survivors of GBV. Lisak and Miller's (2002) findings that most incidences of campus rape are perpetrated by 6 per cent of men reinforced *CSP*'s message that the vast majority of men are not perpetrators but rather bystanders who could take action. *CSP* increased awareness of male survivors by stressing the high incidence of childhood sexual violence (Finkelhor et al. 2005) and including scenarios of same-sex and female-to-male GBV in trainings.

Diverse populations

Recognising the very high incidence of GBV experienced by lesbian, gay, bisexual, transgender, intersex and queer (LGBTIQ) students (Rothman et al. 2011), *CSP* worked with the USM Center for Sexualities and Gender Diversity and DV/SA partner agencies to make materials inclusive, ensure diverse gender and identity representation in programming, and provide student training within the Center.

People with disabilities are at high risk for GBV throughout their lives (Harrell 2014). Conversely, people on the autism spectrum can be challenged to understand social cues, and may inadvertently put themselves at risk of being accused of sexual harassment. The USM Disabilities Service Center was provided with training and partnered in *CSP*'s work.

Approximately 8 per cent of USM's student body is composed of Native Americans, new Americans and international study students. The work of *CSP* was informed by the knowledge that Native women experience the highest rates of sexual violence (Perry 2004), that up to 89 per cent of refugees experience post-traumatic stress disorder (Hollifield et al. 2002), and of differing cultural, social and familial norms around violence. *CSP*, the Multicultural Student Center and the Office of International Programs designed multiple programmes to address the range of needs and interests of these students. For example, the Sisterhood Circle for immigrant women was started and became a safe place for students to discuss sexuality, arranged marriage and other cultural norms they did not feel their American peers understood or respected.

Community-based partners

DV/SA organisations, other nonprofit (charity) legal services programmes and court-based coalitions each brought resources, expertise and perspectives to *CSP*. DV/SA organisations in particular remain critical, providing an important confidential support and reporting option for students, highly trained advocates and educators, and experience of navigating the legal system. *CSP*'s budget included payment for a portion of agency time allowing for consistent campus presence, meetings with survivors and administrators, and presentations and trainings.

Launching prevention education and awareness programming

USM has three campuses: an urban campus serving most of the approximately 9,000 undergraduate and graduate student bodies; a nearby 1,100 student residential campus; and a satellite campus 36 miles (60 kilometres) away. *CSP* piloted programming on the residential campus because it presented:

- students aged 17 to 21, primarily in their first and second years;
- a prevalent drinking culture;
- proximity of off-campus housing for fraternities and athletes;
- Residential Life staff well trained in GBV prevention and response;
- engaged campus police;
- Conduct Office, and Substance Abuse Prevention Program; and,
- Fraternal and sororal student organisations and Athletics Department.

As more than 50 per cent of sexual assaults occur in the first six weeks of the academic year (Krebs et al. 2007), *CSP* focused on orientation and opening weekend events. By year two, *CSP* was presenting at orientations and using theatre programmes *You the Man* (Plourde et al. 2014) and *Speak About It* (Speak About It 2016) to capture interest and efficiently provide information about GBV, consent and being an active bystander. *CSP* later partnered with USM's Theater Department to produce a student-written peer-educational theatre performance about healthy relationships, sexuality and GBV. *Un/Spoken Maine* was performed at orientations on the residential campus and video clips were included in online training.

Although *CSP*'s primary access to students was through non-mandatory, new-student orientations, *CSP* integrated messaging throughout the year into existing awareness efforts and initiated new ways of reaching students by:

- using social media and videos for campus monitors;
- participating in marches and events (e.g. *Take Back the Night* and *Trans Awareness Day*);
- promoting Consent Days which featured sex-positive events, glow-in-the-dark consent T shirts and videos by student leaders;

- presenting in residence and dining halls;
- partnering with Student Activities to include GBV messaging in games, movies and other events;
- co-sponsoring lectures and films with academic departments;
- a service called *Don't Cancel Class* providing presentations for faculty needing class coverage; and,
- targeting identified high-risk groups such as athletic teams and fraternities and sororities.

Athletics, fraternities and sororities

Pre- and post-testing of both the live performances of *Un/Spoken Maine* and the online GBV programme assessed the knowledge base of participating students and pointed to a need for increasing time spent on these issues with residence halls, athletic teams and fraternities. For example, a small subset of incoming male students aged 17 to 19 who answered 'False' to the question 'Alcohol is the number 1 "date rape" drug' also answered 'If someone is sexually assaulted, they are "sometimes" or "always" responsible for the assault.' These responses considered together revealed a lack of awareness of the connection between alcohol and sexual violence, effectively blaming the victim for the crime.

Further complicating cultural shifts on GBV is hook-up culture, defined as 'brief uncommitted sexual encounters between individuals who are not romantic partners or dating one another' (Garcia-Moreno et al. 2012). Hooking up is prevalent on college campuses and the rampant coupling of alcohol and sex encourages misunderstanding at best and assault at worst. In a recent study of sexual behaviour on US campuses it was found that '86.3 per cent of participants portrayed their most recent hook-up experience as one they wanted to have, while 7.6 per cent indicated that their most recent hook-up was an experience they did not want to have or to which they were unable to give consent' (Lewis et al. 2012: 1223). Furthermore, this study found that unwanted and nonconsensual sexual encounters are more likely to occur alongside alcohol and substance use.

The culture of casual sex discourages reporting when sexual assaults occur in this context, as does the close-knit nature of an affiliated group within a larger campus community who may live or socialise together, such as LGBTIQ students, athletic teams or fraternities and sororities (Kimmel 2015).

CSP cultivated allies and strategic partnerships to engage with athletic teams and fraternities and sororities. Residential Life staff members who were athletes or members of fraternities/sororities helped to create opportunities for training and co-sponsoring programming. Early presentations revealed stereotypical views of sexual assault, associating the term only with rape and/or an attack by a stranger on women in 'unsafe' places (dark alley, parking garage), which is counter to data showing that nine of 10 college women know their attacker (Fisher et al. 2000) and attacks are most likely to occur near or at the victim's home (Greenfeld 1997).

Targeting someone at a party, encouraging them to drink large amounts of alcohol, isolating them from their friends and subjecting them to sexual activity is a common scenario on campuses across the US and has been normalised to the degree that it was unrecognised as a crime or a violation by many students.

All fraternities and sororities complete the *Party Program* prior to hosting their first event each year. The *Party Program*'s focus on safety and risk reduction provided an opening for *CSP*, helping make students more aware of the role of alcohol in increasing risk of sexual assault (Abbey 2002). *CSP* also succeeded in institutionalising GBV training for all fraternity and sorority pledges.

Expansion

In year two, initiatives on the residential campus expanded and were adapted for the urban and satellite campuses. Reaching nearly 8,000 additional students posed logistical challenges. The satellite campus was under the jurisdiction of different DV/SA agencies and had not been included in the grant proposal. However, the CC prioritised extending the reach of *CSP* and having DV/SA advocates available to students on all campuses, believing that building a sense of connectedness promotes safety and peer support.

CSP optimised efforts by aligning with other programmes. *CSP* partnered with the suicide prevention programme USM Cares, funded by the National Institutes of Health to train peers to respond to mental health crises. USM Cares staff understood the links between GBV, substance abuse and mental health (Campbell 2002) and expanded the Peer Support curriculum to include GBV messaging. OVW grantee Maine Boys to Men, a local nonprofit organisation focused on healthy masculinity, invited *CSP* to help adapt its *Reducing Sexism and Violence Program* (*RSVP*) for undergraduate participants. *CSP* recruited students to attend the *RSVP* training, which along with USM Cares, helped build a cohort of trained students across the university. Maine Boys to Men also provided funding for *Mentors in Violence Prevention* to train coaches and all autumn and winter athletic teams. This paved the way for a collaborative approach to training athletic teams on mental health, substance abuse, GBV, peer support and bystander intervention.

Outcomes and shortcomings

During year one, following enhanced training of Residential Life staff, reports of sexual assault increased significantly. Reports of dating and domestic abuse took longer to rise. The fact that patterns of abuse occur over time and involve multiple tactics, some of which are subtle and often only occur in private (de Benedictis et al. 2014), may have caused staff and students to overlook them. Similarly, many had not initially recognised stalking behaviour. To increase awareness, *CSP* used technical assistance funds for Michelle Garcia, Director of the National Stalking Resource Center, to provide community-wide training. Over the three-year period there was a notable rise in LGBTIQ student disclosures; however, *CSP* received no reports of female on male GBV. The high number of incidents reported for Clery in 2012 represents the result of the expansion of *CSP* to all USM campuses. The loss of the Coordinator position in June 2013 meant a drop in programming and outreach resulting in a parallel drop in reports.

During the grant period, the CC tracked the number of disclosures from students. With a large commuter student body, most of these incidents were not counted in Clery statistics as they either occurred in the past or off school property. In the autumn of 2011, *CSP* received 18 disclosures; in the spring of 2012 that number rose to 25; and in the autumn of 2012, 57 new disclosures were documented. The case review team confirmed that supports and services were provided to these 57 students including:

- faculty outreach regarding assignments and grades;
- assistance from Financial Aid regarding awards and loans;
- help with housing adjustments, counselling services or conduct options; and
- DV/SA advocacy and support.

Of the 57 students, 83 per cent remained enrolled through the following spring semester, a significant success based on the anecdotal evidence of the high dropout rate of victim/survivors and the relatively low retention rate at the university as a whole.

Following the institution of Conduct Board training, changes to the process to ensure fair and even treatment of both the respondent (accused) and complainant (victim), and increased investigation prior to conduct hearings, outcomes changed dramatically. Nearly all cases brought before the board were found in favour of the complainant, ultimately increasing reporting and trust in the conduct process. *CSP* worked with the Office of Marketing to craft messages showcasing the university's GBV prevention and response as a positive change, in anticipation of questions from the media and prospective parents regarding the jump in Clery statistics.

In summary, the key factors in the increase in reporting over the life of the grant were as follows:

1. dedicated staffing to maintain focus on GBV and advocate for institutionalisation of training and education;
2. the broad reach of the programme in training of students and staff, and raising awareness across the university community;
3. quick response to data indicators to adjust programming to particular populations or issues; and
4. consistent response by employees, the Conduct Office and campus police to incidents of GBV and to cases brought before the Conduct Board.

Several *CSP* initiatives did fall short. *CSP* conducted focus groups on campus climate over the course of the grant; unfortunately, a comprehensive survey was not permitted by the administration. *CSP* planned for universal inclusion of GBV reporting and support information in course syllabi; in-depth training for administrators, faculty and all new employees; and mandatory prevention education for all incoming students. Lacking the administration's support, none of these strategies was enacted and due to budget constraints the position of *CSP* Coordinator was not continued at the conclusion of grant funding in June 2013.

The loss of funding for the Coordinator position dramatically reduced training and awareness efforts, resulting in lower faculty awareness of their reporting role, decreased connection with DV/SA advocates, and fewer in-class presentations, which in turn lowered reports in 2013 and 2014. While university reorganisation has brought stability and consistency back to *CSP* programmes, it will take time to rebuild student and staff awareness and responsiveness.

Since 2013, USM has maintained a consistent use of the response protocol and, like many US universities, has shifted to an investigative model wherein trained Conduct Officers investigate to ascertain what (if any) violation took place and make a determination; this ruling is presented to the complainant and respondent who have the right to appeal to the Conduct Board or ultimately to the Dean of Students or President's designee. The investigative model is seen as more impartial and can resolve cases more quickly, particularly when conducted by an outside entity. In some cases, the process of investigation has encouraged other survivors to come forward, revealing serial offenders. USM's case review team continues to provide oversight and make process adjustments as needed, and a revised GBV policy clarifies that disclosures made at public awareness events such as *Take Back the Night* or candlelight vigils will not trigger a report (University of Maine 2015), helping create an environment of support and change.

USM continues to use live theatre for students at orientations. While a new version of the online orientation training is offered to all students, it is not mandatory and there remains no consequence for students who do not participate out of a concern that such a requirement would deter potential students from enrolling at the university. Anecdotal reports suggest that current students exhibit a higher level of knowledge that sex with someone who is under the influence of alcohol/drugs is sexual assault, and an increase in reports of intimidation and controlling behaviour demonstrates that more students have a deeper understanding of these issues. DV/SA advocates, paid through OVW grant funding, continue to provide awareness programming, educational presentations and training on campus. Their flexibility, skill and ability to relate to the student body have remained valuable to USM and *CSP*.

Recommendations

All *CSP* activities were subject to documentation and regular review, providing the Coordinator with opportunities to reflect on strategies and their impact. In considering these reports and recent research, and with input from current USM staff, the following are practice recommendations for efforts on college campuses to prevent and respond to GBV:

1. create and maintain a diverse body of stakeholders, including student organisations, local service providers, and law enforcement;
2. be guided by good data: annual climate surveys, focus groups, pre- and post-testing, reporting, case outcomes and current research;
3. craft a response protocol that ensures privacy, respects confidentiality, promotes consistent response and includes comprehensive case review;
4. ensure policies and practices are comprehensive, clear and fair;
5. build a shared base of knowledge amongst students and employees, including law enforcement and other stakeholders;
6. use media, arts, activism and events to promote engagement and awareness of support resources;
7. institutionalise GBV education through such mechanisms as new employee orientation and annual notification, mandatory pre-enrollment programming, and course syllabi;
8. give equal education and programming time to domestic and dating violence and stalking as is given to sexual assault and ensure proportionate judicial response;
9. tailor programming to each audience, avoiding a 'one size fits all' approach, and assume the presence of survivors in the room;
10. collaborate with existing programmes and initiatives; and
11. dedicate university (not grant) resources to staffing and maintaining programming.

Shared obstacles

In order to truly change student behaviour, attitudes, and community and campus systems, there are critical issues to be addressed on national and local levels.

Data and efficacy

Most universities use reporting numbers, programme attendance, climate surveys, and pre- and post-testing to measure impact. However, while the level of reporting of GBV is an indication of student awareness of, comfort with and access to reporting, a decrease in reporting does not necessarily indicate a reduction in perpetration.

Staffing

Some universities shortsightedly designate a staff member with little or no training as Title IX Coordinator; others place both GBV prevention and response with one individual, creating responsibilities that are potentially in conflict. Campuses with grant funding often discontinue staff and programming when the funding is complete, undermining project stability and sustainability.

Counting all victims

Lags in acknowledging men as survivors and inconsistencies in data collection hinder change. The 2011 *National Intimate Partner and Sexual Violence Survey* found a surprisingly similar prevalence of nonconsensual sex in the previous 12 months for men and women. This can be explained in part by the survey's recent inclusion of 'being made to penetrate' to the definition of rape, indicating far higher rates of perpetration by females than previously believed or is reported by the media (Stemple and Meyer 2014). Counting all victims will challenge existing GBV prevention and intervention on campuses.

Targeting perpetrators

Earlier findings regarding serial perpetrators (Lisak and Miller 2002) have been challenged by new data finding fewer serial perpetrators and a higher percentage of men perpetrating sexual assault one time early in their college career and not again. The men surveyed attributed the cessation of perpetration to social environment, networks and campus culture. This new data should inform peer education, bystander intervention and other activities that affect campus climate (Swartout et al. 2015).

Judicial response

The suitability of colleges and universities to adjudicate cases of GBV, which would be felonious in a court of law, is still being debated. Lax enforcement of policies and laws governing the use and abuse of alcohol and other substances often undermine messages around the increased risk of sexual assault associated with their use (NIJ 2008). The sexual assault cases most often seen on campuses involve mutual drinking and few witnesses and are unlikely to be accepted for criminal prosecution. However, the preponderance standard used on campuses – that a violation was 'more likely than not' to have occurred – seems incommensurate and while students found responsible for GBV may face expulsion, consequences vary greatly and at most schools the violation will not appear on their transcript.

University accountability

Federal commitment to addressing campus-based GBV is reflected in increased investigation of campuses by the Department of Education Office of Civil Rights (Caplan-Bricker 2016), the passage of the Campus Sexual Violence Elimination Act (USC 2012) and the formation in 2015 of a White House Task Force (United States Government 2016). However, a rush to comply has some universities pushing through policies and programmes that do not provide equal protections to all parties (Bazelon 2015) and even purchasing expensive commercially available programmes that are not evidence-based (Nelson 2015). Federally sanctioned programmes in bystander intervention (Banyard et al. 2014) are promoted, yet other research-based strategies such as empowerment self-defence (see Chapter 7), which provides participants with the awareness and verbal and physical skills to increase their own safety and avoid or interrupt an attack, are not (Senn et al. 2015).

Conclusion

The cost of not addressing GBV can be astronomical for universities facing civil lawsuits and potential loss of funding following federal investigation. Yet it is this financial threat, coupled with consistent pressure from student activists, which continues to prompt dramatic change on campuses across the US. Since the White House launched a web programme, *It's On Us* (2015), to engage student activism around campus assault in 2015, a quarter of a million people have taken the *It's On Us* pledge and hundreds of events have been sponsored on campuses nationwide. Other web-based programmes created by student activists such as *End Rape on Campus* and *Know Your IX* have been instrumental in making information on federal regulations governing campus response, ways to assess university policies and file a complaint, and effective activist tactics widely available to students. These groups and others have effectively kept pressure on federal and state governments and universities to strengthen laws and policies and support survivors. *Campus Safety Project*'s commitment to strengthening relationships and challenging the status quo to build sustainable change created a strong foundation for this work at USM and is a powerful example of an effective approach to addressing GBV on campuses nationwide.

References

Abbey, A. (2002) 'Alcohol-related sexual assault: a common problem among college students', *Journal of Studies on Alcohol Supplement*, 14: 118–28.

Banyard, V.L., Moynihan, M.M., Cares, A.C. and Warner, R.A. (2014) 'How do we know if it works? Defining measurable outcomes in bystander-focused violence prevention', *Psychology of Violence*, 4(1): 101–15.

Bazelon, E. (2015) 'The return of sex wars: the decades-old intellectual debate simmering beneath the current conversation over sexual assault on campus', *New York Times Magazine*. Online. Available at www.nytimes.com (accessed 10 September 2015).

Campbell, C.J. (2002) 'Health consequences of intimate partner violence', *The Lancet*, 359: 1331–6.

Caplan-Bricker, N. (2016) 'An important new tool in the crackdown against sexual assault', *Slate.com*. Online. Available at www.slate.com/blogs/xx_factor/2016/01/11/an_important_new_tool_in_the_crackdown_against_campus_sexual_assault.html (accessed 11 January 2016).

de Benedictis, T., Jaffe, J. and Segal, J. (2014) 'Domestic violence and abuse: types, signs, symptoms, causes, and effects', *American Academy of Experts in Traumatic Stress*. Online. Available at www.aaets.org/article144.htm (accessed 16 January 2016).

Finkelhor, D., Ormrod, R.K., Turner, H.A. and Hamby, S.L. (2005) 'The victimization of children and youth: a comprehensive, national survey', *Child Maltreatment*, 10(1): 5–25.

Fisher, B.S., Cullen F.T. and Turner M.G. (2000) *The Sexual Victimization of College Women*, Washington, DC: National Institute of Justice and the Bureau of Justice Statistics. Online. Available at http://ncjrs.gov/pdffiles1/nij/182369.pdf (accessed 14 March 2017).

Garcia-Moreno, C., Guedes, A. and Knerr, W. (2012) *Understanding and Addressing Violence against Women: health consequences*, Geneva: World Health Organization. Online. Available at http://apps.who.int/iris/bitstream/10665/77431/1/WHO_RHR_12.43_eng.pdf (accessed 10 January 2015).

Greenfeld, L.A. (1997) *1997 Sex Offenses and Offenders Study*, US Department of Justice, Bureau of Statistics. Online. Available at http://bjs.gov/content/pub/pdf/SOO.PDF (accessed 10 December 2015).

Harrell, E. (2014) *Crime against People with Disabilities, 2009–2012: Statistical Tables*, Washington, DC: US Department of Justice Office of Justice Programs Bureau of Justice Statistics. Online. Available at www.bjs.gov/content/pub/pdf/capd0912st.pdf (accessed 15 January 2016).

Hollifield, M., Warner, T.D., Lian, N., Krakow, B., Jenkins, J.H., Kesler, J., Stevenson, J. and Westermeyer, J. (2002) 'Measuring trauma and health status in refugees: a critical review', *Journal of the American Medical Association*, 288: 611–21.

It's On Us (2015) *itsonus.org*. Online. Available at http://itsonus.org/ (accessed 10 September 2015).

Kimmel, M. (2015) 'A recipe for sexual assault', *The Atlantic*. Online. Available at www.theatlantic.com/education/archive/2015/08/what-makes-a-campus-rape-prone/402065/ (accessed 16 September 2015).

Krebs, C.P., Lindquist, C.H., Warner, T.D., Fisher, B.S. and Martin, S.L. (2007) *The Campus Sexual Assault (CSA) Study*, Washington, DC: National Institute of Justice. Online. Available at www.ncjrs.gov/pdffiles1/nij/grants/221153.pdf (accessed 10 September 2015).

Kretzmann, J. and McKnight, J. (1993) *Building Communities from the Inside Out: a path toward finding and mobilizing a community's assets*, Chicago: ACTA Publications.

Krug, E.G., Mercy, J.A., Dahlberg, L.L., Zwi, A.B. and Lozano, R. (2002) *World Report on Violence and Health*, Geneva: World Health Organization.

Lewis, M.A., Granato, H., Blayney, J.A., Lostutter, T.W. and Kilmer, J.R. (2012) 'Predictors of hooking up sexual behaviors and emotional reactions among US college students', *Archives of Sexual Behavior*, 41: 1219–29.

Lisak, D. and Miller, P. (2002) 'Repeat rape and multiple offending among undetected rapists', *Violence and Victims*, 17(1): 73–84.

McMahon, S., Stepleton, K., O'Connor, J. and Cusano, J. (2015) *Campus Climate Surveys: lessons learned from the Rutgers–New Brunswick pilot assessment*, New Brunswick: Rutgers School of Social Work. Online. Available at http://socialwork.rutgers.edu/Libraries/VAWC/Rutgers_Campus_Climate_Assessment_Process_-Final_Report.sflb.ashx (accessed 10 September 2015).

Nelson, E. (2015) 'To comply with new sexual assault prevention requirements, colleges turn to online courses', *Star Tribune* (Minneapolis, MN), 7 September.

NIJ (National Institute of Justice) (2008) *Alcohol Use Increases the Risk of Sexual Assault*. Online. Available at www.nij.gov/topics/crime/rape-sexual-violence/campus/pages/alcohol.aspx (accessed 10 December 2015).

Perry, S.W. (2004) *American Indians and Crime: a BJS statistical profile 1992–2002*, Washington, DC: US Department of Justice, Office of Justice Programs Bureau of Justice Statistics. Online. Available at www.justice.gov/sites/default/files/otj/docs/american_indians_and_crime.pdf (accessed 10 December 2015).

Plourde, C., Taket, A., Murray, V. and van der Werf, P. (2014) 'The development of a brief theatre-based programme for the promotion of bystander engagement and violence prevention', *Journal of Applied Arts and Health*, 5: 377–92.

Rothman, E., Deinera, E. and Baughman, A. (2011) 'The prevalence of sexual assault against people who identify as gay, lesbian, or bisexual in the United States: a systematic review', *Trauma, Violence and Abuse*, 12: 55–66.

Senn, C.Y., Eliasziw, M., Barata, P.C., Thurston, W.E., Newby-Clark, I.R., Radtke, H.L. and Hobden, K.L. (2015) 'Efficacy of a sexual assault resistance program for university women', *New England Journal of Medicine*, 372: 2326–35.

Speak About It (2016) *About the Show*. Online. Available at http://speakaboutitonline.com/about (accessed 24 June 2016).

Stemple, L. and Meyer, I.H. (2014) 'The sexual victimization of men in America: new data challenge old assumptions', *American Journal of Public Health*, 104(6): e19–26.

Swartout, K.M., Koss, M.P., White, J.W., Thompson, M.P., Abbey, A. and Bellis, A.L. (2015) 'Trajectory analysis of the campus serial rapist assumption', *Journal of the American Medical Association Pediatrics*, 169: 1148–54.

United States Government (2016) *Not Alone: together against sexual assault*. Online. Available at www.notalone.gov (accessed 24 June 2016).

University of Maine (2015) *Sex Discrimination, Sexual Harassment, Sexual Assault, Relationship Violence, Stalking and Retaliation: University of Maine system policies and procedures*, University of Maine. Online. Available at https://umaine.edu/eo/policies-procedures/sex-discrimination-sexual-harassment-sexual-assault-relationship-violence-stalking-and-retaliation/ (accessed 10 December 2015).

USC (United States Congress) (1994) *H.R.3355 Violent Crime Control and Law Enforcement Act of 1994: Title IV*. Online. Available at www.congress.gov/bill/103rd-congress/house-bill/3355 (accessed 10 January 2016).

USC (United States Congress) (2012) *Campus Sexual Violence Elimination Act*. Online. Available at www.congress.gov/bill/112th-congress/house-bill/2016 (accessed 16 September 2015).

USDOE OCR (United States Department of Education Office for Civil Rights) (2011) *Dear Colleague Letter*. Online. Available at www2.ed.gov/about/offices/list/ocr/letters/colleague-201109.html (accessed 10 September 2015).

USDOJ (United States Department of Justice) (2015) *Overview of Title IX of the Educational Amendments of 1972, 20 U.S.C. A§ 1681 ET. SEQ*. Online. Available at www.justice.gov/crt/overview-title-ix-education-amendments-1972-20-usc-1681-et-seq (accessed 16 September 2015).

USM (University of Southern Maine) (2016) *Campus Safety Project: information for USM employees*. Online. Available at https://usm.maine.edu/sites/default/files/campussafety-project/CSP_Staff%20Brochure_R2.pdf (accessed 24 June 2016).

Ward, D. and Mann J.L. (2011) *The Handbook for Campus Safety and Security Reporting*, Washington, DC: US Department of Education Office of Postsecondary Education. Online. Available at www2.ed.gov/admins/lead/safety/handbook.pdf (accessed 10 December 2015).

Woods, T.O. (2000) *First Response to Victims of Crime: a handbook for law enforcement officers on how to approach and help*, Washington, DC: US Department of Justice Office of Justice Programs Office for Victims of Crime. Online. Available at www.ncjrs.gov/ovc_archives/reports/firstrep/welcome.html (accessed 14 January 2016).

7

PREVENTION, RESISTANCE, RECOVERY, REVOLUTION

Feminist empowerment self-defence

Lynne Marie Wanamaker

Introduction

The problem of preventing sexual and gender-based violence rests on a paradox. On the one hand, individuals who perpetrate violence are singularly responsible for the harm they deliver, and therefore have the greatest power and moral obligation to end it. On the other hand, those most negatively affected – those at elevated risk of assault, those who have been hurt before, and their allies – can take action to increase safety for themselves and others. This has been called the 'self-defence paradox'.

Empowerment self-defence (ESD) responds to this paradox. ESD elevates the agency of women and others at risk of victimisation through skills for identifying, avoiding, interrupting, responding to and mitigating the effects of sexual violence. Arising from the feminist grassroots movement as an activist response to sexual and gendered violence, ESD has matured into a cogent, comprehensive methodology. In the past several decades, researchers have amassed an evidence base affirming the efficacy of ESD in preventing assault and delivering ancillary benefits to both never-victimised women and to survivors of sexual assault (Brecklin 2008; Hollander 2014; Sarnquist et al. 2014; Senn et al. 2015). Self-defence has been recommended by trauma experts as both a prevention strategy and an intervention with survivors of violence (Herman 1997; van der Kolk 2006). Proponents of ESD contend that it addresses the root causes of sexual and gender-based violence by challenging oppressive gender norms and social stereotypes (McCaughey and Cermele 2015; Ullman 2007), and contributes to the anti-violence movement by promoting an understanding of violence within a social context, elevating women and girls as 'powerful and effective social change agents', while holding those who perpetrate accountable for the harm they deliver (Thompson 2014: 351). In light of the fact that little data exists to demonstrate the efficacy of prevention interventions

(Ellsberg et al. 2015), ESD is an important and innovative intervention that could prevent countless acts of violence against women and girls worldwide.

What is empowerment self-defence?

ESD is a group-based intervention that delivers skills to address a continuum of interpersonal violations, from verbal harassment to sexual, physical and life-threatening assault. It is characterised by an explicitly survivor-centred ethos that holds perpetrators solely responsible for sexual violence and rejects cultural victim-blaming. ESD instructors stress that 'there is nothing any survivor could do or not do that could "cause" a sexual assault, harassment, intimate partner violence, or stalking to happen' (Taylor and Wanamaker 2014).

ESD is informed by the reality that known-assailant violence is significantly more prevalent than stranger assault (WHO 2014). Accordingly, ESD instruction includes education about the earliest warning signs of interpersonal and relationship violence, characteristics of healthy relationships, and communication skills for negotiating sexual consent or establishing personal boundaries. Classes include opportunities to practise assessment and verbal skills for identifying, interrupting or de-escalating violent situations.

ESD classes examine how culture and socialisation may disadvantage women and others at elevated risk of victimisation from being able to trust or act upon their instincts regarding interpersonal safety. In contrast to Ullman's observation that 'rape is typically presented as a personal problem and almost never presented in socio-political terms that emphasise disparate power relations or structural causes (e.g. gender inequity)' (Ullman 2010: 24), ESD directly addresses the social construction of gender norms and systems of power and privilege, and provides skill-based opportunities to unlearn gender socialisation (Rozee and Koss 2001).

Among the strategies ESD instructors employ for disrupting gender norms is the still radical act of teaching women to fight. ESD teaches physical defence techniques that are simple to learn and effective when other options have been exhausted. The subset of practical self-protection skills taught in ESD may be derivative of but are distinct from stylised or traditional martial arts (Senn et al. 2015; Thompson 2014). Though early feminist self-defence stressed the importance of women-only spaces (Brecklin 2008; Searles and Berger 1987), a more modern understanding of gender, recognition of the elevated risk of interpersonal violence experienced by transgender people and a desire to engage men as supportive allies has led some ESD providers to reevaluate their orientation to gender separatism. Finally, ESD encourages connection to healing and community organising resources to recover from violence and increase safety for all people.

This working definition establishes ESD as distinct from other forms of self-defence, many of which reproduce victim-blaming cultural beliefs and recommend as self-protective tactics which are not associated with reducing sexual violence and which compromise women's autonomy. Searles and Berger (1987: 62) characterised such advice as encouraging women 'to limit their mobility and to depend upon men, large barking dogs, chemical sprays, whistles, and other external agents for their protection'. Nearly thirty years later, Schorn's (2015) analysis of 'the terrible manual cops use to teach "rape prevention"' revealed that one of the highest profile self-defence programmes in the US continues to perpetuate the same 'fear based, patriarchal' misinformation. Rape Aggression Defence, taught by police officers across the nation and ubiquitous on college campuses, acknowledges that it is not intended for use in known-assailant assaults, and provides a catalogue of detailed 'life-restricting' recommendations.

If gender-based violence is not only a public health issue but also a violation of human rights, prevention interventions which restrict the behaviour of those affected must be considered a further abrogation of rights. ESD advocates and researchers stress that unlike inferior forms of self-defence and other victim-focused interventions, ESD empowers women with information, options and skills (Hollander 2014; Rozee and Koss 2001; Thompson 2014). Thompson (2014: 253) notes, 'the failure to differentiate police and traditional martial arts self-defense programmes from feminist or empowering self-defense training limits the ability of feminist self-defense organisations to be an integral part of the anti-violence movement'.

ESD prevents sexual assault

Increasingly, rigorous evaluation demonstrates that ESD effectively prevents sexual assault. Recent studies build on earlier, qualitative evidence by imposing experimental and quasi-experimental designs to determine the impact of ESD training on an individual's subsequent risk of sexual violence. Three studies in particular reflect this emerging evidence.

In a mixed-method study of a 10-week, university-based feminist self-defence class, Hollander (2014) used a quasi-experimental design to assess the effectiveness of ESD one year post-training. ESD-trained women reported not only fewer and less severe completed assaults than similar women in a comparison group, but also reported fewer attempted assaults. This was notable because it might be reasonable to anticipate that women trained in self-defence, with enhanced awareness of the definitions and patterns of sexual assault, would be more likely to label unwelcome sexual contact as an assault. The author suggests that the self-protective action promoted through ESD training may occur early in an assault trajectory, interrupting the violation before it escalates to the level of assault. Although this quasi-experimental study design was limited by the absence of random assignment to the intervention or comparison groups, it improved on previous studies by utilising a one-year follow-up. Statistical analyses controlled for differences between the students who received ESD training and a comparison group of female students recruited from unrelated academic courses. The analysis supported the conclusion that the ESD intervention effectively reduced rates of sexual assault, including sexual contact, sexual coercion, and attempted and completed rape. At one year, none of the ESD-trained women (n=75) had experienced a completed rape, in contrast to 3 per cent of the comparison group (n=183).

In a randomised controlled trial (RCT) of 1,978 adolescent girls in Nairobi, Kenya, Sarnquist et al. (2014) found that the sexual assault rate among ESD-trained girls decreased from 18 to 11 per 100 person years, with no change in the control group. This intervention provided twelve hours of empowerment, de-escalation and self-defence skills; those in the control group received a life-skills class. Sexual assault rates were measured at 10.5 months post-intervention. ESD-trained girls reported using the skills they learned to prevent both physical assault (52 per cent of retained participants reporting this result) and harassment (65 per cent reporting). Results indicate that the girls used primarily verbal skills (45 per cent of those who interrupted assault, 59 per cent of those who interrupted harassment); a combination of verbal and physical skills (29 per cent assault, 26 per cent harassment); or physical skills alone (25 per cent assault, 15 per cent harassment). This study was limited by the fact that randomisation occurred on the community, rather than on the individual level, and that it relied on self-report as the primary measure of outcomes. While baseline similarities were ensured between the intervention and comparison groups, hidden differences may have influenced outcomes. Nevertheless, these findings indicate that the skills delivered through ESD are flexible, effective and relevant to a range of scenarios.

In another RCT of Canadian first-year university women, Senn and colleagues (2015) found that the one-year risk of completed rape among self-defence-trained women (n=451) was 46 per cent lower than in a control group (n=442). The one-year risk of attempted rape was 63 per cent lower. Notably, the effect of the intervention was not significantly affected by previous victimisation, despite significant differences within the control group: the one-year risk of completed rape among previously victimised members of the control group was nearly four times as high as for those with no previous victimisation.

Students in the intervention group received the *Enhanced Assess, Acknowledge, Act Sexual Assault Resistance (Enhanced AAA)* programme; those in the control group received brochures about sexual assault, in keeping with the universities' standard sexual assault-prevention education. *AAA* is consistent with ESD principles and delivers skills regarding assessment of risk, problem-solving, acknowledging danger from known assailants, overcoming internal barriers to resistance, and response to verbal coercion, as well as physical defence and fighting skills. *Enhanced AAA* integrates these competencies with content adapted from the *Our Whole Lives* sexuality education (Senn et al. 2015). The Sexuality and Relationships component of *Enhanced AAA* delivers sexual information and terminology and provides a context for exploring sexual attitudes and values and practising sexual communication. This study improved on previous efforts to integrate emancipatory sexuality education into the *AAA* curriculum (Senn et al. 2011) by increasing the number of training hours and the volume of practice opportunities and by devoting increased attention to escalating resistance/defensive responses to a perpetrator's persistence (Senn et al. 2015). The study utilised open-label recruitment/enrolment, resulting in higher rates of previous victimisation among the sample than would be anticipated in random sampling. The study was further limited by the impossibility of blinding assignment to the intervention and control groups, and by the reliance on self-report of victimisation. The researchers note that the incentive and retention structures specific to the study protocol may have contributed to the achievement of high adherence rates (91 per cent in the intervention group). Nevertheless, this study delivers strong evidence of ESD's effectiveness with both previously victimised and non-previously victimised first-year university women. In the US this population is considered to be at elevated risk of sexual violence and has been the focus of significant public policy attention coordinated through the White House Task Force to Protect Students from Sexual Assault (Obama 2014).

The findings of these studies assessing ESD are all the more powerful when considered in the broader context of prevention research. Despite significant attention to the issue of sexual and gendered violence in activist, legal, social service and public health sectors in the US and internationally over the past forty years, few interventions have been identified to effectively reduce perpetrator behaviour (DeGue et al. 2014; Ellsberg et al. 2015) or rape prevalence (Hollander 2014; Rozee and Koss 2001). Ellsberg et al. (2015) conducted a systematic review on the efficacy of interventions to reduce many types of violence against women and girls falling both within and outside the scope of ESD. Having examined 84 rigorously evaluated (experimental or quasi-experimental designs) studies and an additional 58 reviews, the authors concluded that the evidence base disproportionately represents high-income countries, with the US accounting for two-thirds of the intervention studies. Among the high-income-country studies, most have addressed intimate partner violence, followed by non-partner sexual assault, and have assessed the efficacy of response rather than prevention interventions.

DeGue et al. (2014: 346), whose review of rigorously evaluated primary prevention strategies for sexual violence perpetration informed the policy recommendations of the United States White House Task Force to Protect Students from Sexual Assault, concluded that overall there exists a 'dearth of effective prevention strategies'. The paucity of promising results was exacerbated by the exclusion of ESD efficacy studies from consideration. This exclusion rests on the categorisation of ESD as 'risk reduction' rather than 'primary prevention' within a public health model. Risk reduction interventions are intended to prevent victimisation whereas primary prevention is defined as stopping violence before it occurs by reducing perpetration behaviour. Arguably this is a false dichotomy: the categorisation of ESD as risk reduction rather than primary prevention rests on whether identical actions are taken by a woman on her own behalf or by a third party in order to protect her. In this way, the elevation of perpetrator-only solutions may have the unwelcome consequence of promoting individual and cultural beliefs about women's vulnerability to assault and incapacity for defensive actions (McCaughey and Cermele 2015).

ESD delivers ancillary benefits

Findings indicative of ESD's efficacy in reducing individuals' risk of sexual violence are further contextualised by evidence that the intervention delivers benefits to students' wellbeing. ESD-trained students in Hollander's (2014) study reported increases in confidence in their own ability to defend against assault. These changes were sustained at one-year follow-up. An earlier examination of both basic and enhanced *AAA* also found significant positive effects on students' self-efficacious beliefs in their own capacity to defend themselves (Senn et al. 2011). Sarnquist et al. (2014) noted that ESD-trained adolescents who did experience sexual assault were more likely to disclose the incidents than those in the control group, enabling them to access supportive services.

These findings join previous research attesting to both psychological and behavioural benefits of ESD, including a review of 20 published and non-published evaluations of women's self-defence classes conducted by Brecklin (2008). Improvements were shown in assertiveness, perceived control, self-efficacy and physical competence and reductions in anxiety and helplessness. Mixed results were found with regard to self-esteem, perceived control and fear. Brecklin drew a distinction between 'participatory' and 'avoidance' behaviours, the former described as behaviours reflecting 'freedom of movement' (Brecklin 2008: 71) and the latter as self-limiting behaviours intended to reduce victimisation risk. Across the studies included in Brecklin's review that measured these outcomes, improvements were shown in participatory behaviours and mixed results were found in avoidance behaviours. These findings affirm the distinction between empowering self-protective action (for example, assessing an environment or interaction for signs of danger) and restricting self-protective actions (for example, not walking alone after dark).

ESD is consistent with what works to interrupt rape

Findings regarding the efficacy of ESD training to reduce an individual's risk of violence are also contextualised in research regarding the effectiveness of rape resistance and self-protective action. ESD advocates have distinguished between *learning* self-defence and *using* self-defence to defend oneself in an assault scenario (McCaughey and Cermele 2015). Outcome evaluations of self-defence instruction interventions largely represent the former, by measuring the effect of having attended self-defence training on a student's subsequent risk of assault. Evidence also indicates that using self-defence – employing defensive action on one's own behalf during an assault – is also effective in reducing the risk of completed rape.

In a comprehensive examination of victim protective action in a large probability sample (n=2,011) of sexual assaults drawn from the *National Crime Victimization Survey, 1992–2002*, Tark and Kleck (2014) determined that most self-protective actions reduce the risk of rape completion without significantly increasing the risk of additional injury. This research improved on previous studies of women's resistance actions by taking into account the sequence of the self-protective actions and any injuries to the intended victim. Data analysis demonstrated that protective action is rarely followed by increased or serious injury. This work disproves the common assumption and argument against self-defence that fighting back increases a woman's risk of additional harm and led the authors to state emphatically:

> We believe these findings imply that any police officers and rape victim support groups who counsel against forceful resistance should reconsider these policies. The notion that resistance increases the victim's chances of additional injury beyond the rape itself is not supported by the data.
>
> *(Tark and Kleck 2014: 290)*

The tactics found by Tark and Kleck (2014) to be most effective in interrupting assaults, which were found to decrease the risk of rape completion 80–86 per cent, were largely consistent with ESD teaching. They included distancing and fleeing strategies such as running away, calling for help or otherwise attracting assistance, physically struggling, and unarmed strikes and blows to the rapist. This is consistent with Ullman's (2007) findings that fighting back, fleeing and yelling or screaming are associated with reduced odds of completed rape. Notably, the *AAA Sexual Assault Resistance Program* developed and evaluated by Senn et al. (2015) was informed by Ullman's research regarding effective self-protective strategies during assault situations.

ESD contributes to women's capacity to fight back in assault situations in several ways. First, ESD training helps women to accurately identify situations in which they are at risk of assault, and to respond rapidly and with an appropriate level of intensity. This is achieved by accurately reflecting the elevated risk of known-assailant versus stranger assaults, by delivering information about behaviours that may precede or indicate the potential for sexual violence, and by providing opportunities to practise assessment and intervention skills. Second, ESD increases women's belief that they will be successful if they do employ defensive skills. Finally, ESD increases women's physical competence and fighting skills.

ESD offers benefits to survivors

ESD's uniquely survivor-sensitive and trauma-informed approach responds to the reality that prevention of sexual violence and response/intervention with survivors are functionally indivisible. This is suggested by a life-course perspective and supported by evidence indicating that, once victimised, individuals are at elevated risk of repeated sexual violence. Data from the US Centers for Disease Control and Prevention's (CDC's) *National Intimate Partner and Sexual Violence Survey (NISVS) 2010* reveals that individuals who reported a first rape when they were younger than 18 had a higher prevalence of rape as adults (Black et al. 2011). The 2010 *NISVS* also reveals that most sexual violations occur early in the life course: nearly 80 per cent of female victims of completed rape reported that their first victimisation occurred before age 25; more than 40 per cent before age 18. Functionally, this suggests that it is realistic to expect that survivors will be present throughout populations and that any community-level prevention initiatives must anticipate their participation. This data also identifies survivors of sexual violence as a high-risk group who may benefit from targeted prevention interventions, and identifies revictimisation as a potential negative sequela of initial victimisation. Nevertheless, there is little indication that response interventions successful at mitigating other negative effects of victimisation (e.g. physical and mental health outcomes) reduce the risk of re-victimisation (Ellsberg et al. 2015).

Because ESD instructors anticipate the presence of survivors in all classes, they have developed a robust practice wisdom to facilitate the participation of individuals who have experienced sexual and gendered violence. The foundation of these practices is the articulate and proactive repudiation of victim-blaming and other social phenomena – such as rape denial, myths, stereotypes and negative social responses – which Ullman describes as the scaffolding of a 'rape-supportive environment' (Ullman 2010: 14). The National Women's Martial Arts Federation (NWMAF), a US-based international certifying body of self-defence instructors in the ESD model, has included trauma-related professional development content in its annual instructor certification conference since 2008. NWMAF-certified self-defence instructors are required to affirm their agreement with a set of survivor-centred assumptions developed by the (now defunct) National Coalition against Sexual Assault's ad-hoc committee on self-defence.

Philosophical assumptions developed by the National Coalition against Sexual Assault (NCASA) self-defense ad-hoc Committee regarding the teaching of self-defense:

a.   Women do not ask for, cause, invite, or deserve to be assaulted. Women and men sometimes exercise poor judgment about safety behavior, but that does not make them responsible for the attack. Attackers are responsible for their attacks and their use of violence to overpower, control and abuse another human being.

b.   Whatever a woman's decision in a given self-defense situation, whatever action she does or does not take, she is not at fault. A woman's decision to survive the best way she can must be respected. Self-defense classes should not be used as judgment against a victim/survivor.

c.   Good self-defense programs do not 'tell' an individual what she 'should' or 'should not' do. A program should offer options, techniques, and a way of analyzing situations. A program may point out what USUALLY works best in MOST situations, but each situation is unique and the final decision rests with the person actually confronted by the situation.

d.   Empowerment is the goal of a good self-defense program. The individual's right to make decisions about her participation must be respected. Pressure should not be brought to bear in any way to get a woman to participate in an activity if she is hesitant or unwilling.

Source: CALCASA (California Coalition against Sexual Assault) 1999: 401.

ESD instructors demonstrate this philosophical orientation through specific practice behaviours described by the NWMAF (Gregory et al. 2015) as core competencies. Whether responding to general discussion of sexual violence or disclosures within the classroom, ESD instructors indicate belief in survivors, validate their choices and avoid questioning their decisions. This elevation of individual agency is echoed in classroom management. NWMAF-certified instructors are expected to utilise an opt-in, consent model that empowers students to determine their own level of participation. Instructors do not touch students' bodies without permission and instruction is provided on how to refuse touch. In these ways, the ESD classroom becomes a laboratory within which survivors can practise asserting agency and regain empowerment. ESD instructors are also expected to develop skills for responding to disclosures and trauma responses which may arise in the classroom, and to model supportive and empathic responses.

Some authors distinguish between self-defence classes offered specifically for survivors and those open to more general populations (Brecklin 2008; Rosenblum and Taska 2014), and some ESD providers include such classes among their offerings. However, the significant number of survivors throughout the population, and the fact that many survivors may not self-identify as a condition of enrolling in a self-defence class, support the integration of survivor-centred practice throughout all programmes.

In addition to practice behaviours and teaching strategies specifically intended to disrupt rape-supportive culture and cultivate a survivor-supportive learning environment, aspects intrinsic to ESD may also be of particular benefit to survivors of sexual violence. For example, ESD students are encouraged to use awareness of environmental cues and their own instinctive fear response, in combination with new knowledge regarding behavioural predictors of interpersonal violence, to cultivate skills for avoiding, interrupting and/or neutralising danger (Thompson 2014). Emerging research with individuals with post-traumatic stress disorder (PTSD) suggests that this type of experience may contribute to recovery by increasing tolerance of physical sensations (van der Kolk et al. 2014). Trauma expert Bessel van der Kolk and his colleagues (2014) suggest that increased tolerance of the physical sensations of the fear response not only contributes to survivors' post-traumatic recovery but also provides the opportunity to use those physical signals to identify dangerous situations. This could increase a survivor's odds of successfully avoiding, interrupting or defending against re-victimisation.

Emerging research also suggests that mind–body practices may be effective in improving outcomes for trauma survivors (Kim et al. 2013; Rosenblum and Taska 2014; van der Kolk 2006; van der Kolk et al. 2014). While ESD should not be considered a responsive or clinical intervention, it shares some attributes with these somatic practices. By definition, ESD, including the highly successful programmes evaluated by Hollander (2014), Sarnquist et al. (2014) and Senn et al. (2015), utilises interaction, movement, skills practice and participation. These behaviours are also congruous with recommendations for 'active coping', considered beneficial for trauma survivors (LeDeux and Gorman 2001). Notably, these instructional practices are also more consistent with 'best practices' in prevention, which recommend utilisation of a variety of instructional methods, than many other prevention interventions (DeGue et al. 2014).

Finally, the ESD classroom provides survivors with a unique opportunity for connection with others. Disruption of interpersonal attachment is considered to be one of the most salient consequences of sexual trauma and reconnection essential to healing and recovery (Herman 1997; van der Kolk 2006). The opt-in nature of ESD instruction allows survivors to control their participation within the group, which may make it an easier or more successful social context to navigate. ESD instructors' capacity to normalise emotional responses and model and promote emotional regulation skills supports survivors' participation. Qualitative research (non-survivor-specific) indicates that self-defence classes are experienced by participants as supportive and beneficial (Brecklin and Middendorf 2014). The supportive ESD environment may also be reparative for survivors who did not experience social support during or following victimisation (Rosenbloom and Taska 2014).

ESD operates at multiple levels of impact

Since its inception, the feminist self-defence movement has articulated a connection between individual experiences of victimisation and cultural support for violence, and between individual self-protection and collective social change. In current practice, ESD continues to illuminate how cultural norms may disadvantage women from being able to trust or act upon their instincts regarding interpersonal safety, and how socialisation may undermine women's readiness to interrupt and defend against interpersonal violation (Hollander 2014; Rozee and Koss 2001). ESD shares the characteristic of directly addressing social norms supportive of sexual violence and gender inequity with other types of sexual violence prevention programming found to be successful in low- and middle-income countries (Ellsberg et al. 2015).

Consideration of the cultural context of sexual violence invites examination of structural causes including inequities in access to power, privilege, opportunities and resources (Thompson 2014). Many ESD instructors extend their socio-political analysis of sexual and gendered violence to considering the intersections of systems of oppression. For example, NWMAF encourages cultural competence and effective cross-cultural work (Trembath et al. 2015). Political awareness and consideration of violence within the forces of sexism, racism, classism and other systems of oppression is considered a core competency for NWMAF-certified instructors (Gregory et al. 2015).

ESD advocates contend that women's development of physical defensive skills – what Thompson (2014: 354) terms 'the centrality of embodiment' in ESD practice – undermines personal and social beliefs about men's physical superiority, women's vulnerability, and the inevitability of sexual violence. This stands in stark contrast to violence-prevention strategies which invoke protection of women by third parties, such as the United States' White House Task Force to *Protect* Students from Sexual Assault (emphasis added) or the promotion of bystander intervention over self-defence. McCaughey and Cermele (2015) have gone so far as to claim that the routine exclusion of self-defence from campus-based rape prevention in the US constitutes a 'hidden curriculum' which reinforces cultural norms, vis-a-vis the gender status quo, that support rape.

Social norms associating violence with masculinity leave many women ignorant of the mechanics of physical fighting and reluctant to use their bodies 'as physically powerful instruments of action' (Rozee and Koss 2001: 298). In addition to informing women that specific defensive action such as struggling, striking, running away and calling for help reduce the risk of rape completion (Tark and Kleck 2014), ESD classes provide an opportunity to practise effective physical techniques. Experiencing one's own body as strong, powerful and potentially damaging, and witnessing other women as physically powerful, not only cultivates individual self-efficacy; it also undermines cultural systems of belief regarding men's invincibility (Thompson 2014). Ullman extends this thinking when she reflects that women's individual resistance to sexual violence has the potential to send a collective message:

> If women fought back, perhaps there would be fewer rapists who thought they could so easily get away with it. While resistance would not completely stop rape or rapists, perhaps it would give them pause and show them that women would no longer 'take it lying down,' so to speak.
>
> *(Ullman 2010: 345)*

ESD advocates argue that the verbal and assertiveness skills practised in ESD alter women's presentation and behaviour, potentially challenging gender norms and perceptions about female vulnerability. Veteran ESD instructor Susan Schorn writes about communication skills as:

> critical to transformation of all kinds: personal, interpersonal, political . . . When I teach, I spend at least a quarter of every class on the concept of 'Yell' – that's how vital it is to empowerment and safety. Yelling is the opposite of silencing. Yelling stands at the very heart of feminism.
>
> *(Schorn 2014)*

Women trained in ESD are more confident of their ability to defend themselves, and more accurate in their assessment of the threat of sexual violence. By countering systemic misinformation – regarding the relative risk of stranger versus known-assailant violence, the effectiveness of self-protective action, men's physical invincibility, women's physical vulnerability and the inevitability of women's sexual violation – ESD disrupts rape mythology and fears that limit women's freedom of movement and social engagement (Rozee and Koss 2001). Advocates argue that this changes how women carry themselves throughout their lives, and not only in the acute danger of an assault. As ESD instructors Taylor and Wanamaker write:

> Women who have taken empowerment self-defense interact differently with the men in their lives. They take more healthy risks. They live more authentically. They raise their children differently. And on and on.
>
> *(Taylor and Wanamaker 2014)*

References

Black, M.C., Basile, K.C., Breiding, M.J., Smith, S.G., Walters, M.L., Merrick, M.T., Chen, J. and Stevens, M.R. (2011) *The National Intimate Partner and Sexual Violence Survey (NISVS): 2010 summary report*, Atlanta: GA: National Center for Injury Prevention and Control, Centers for Disease Control and Prevention. Online. Available at www.cdc.gov/violenceprevention/pdf/nisvs_report2010-a.pdf (accessed 22 December 2015).

Brecklin, L.R. (2008) 'Evaluation outcomes of self-defense training for women: a review', *Aggression and Violent Behavior*, 13: 60–76.

Brecklin, L.R. and Middendorf, R.K. (2014) 'The group dynamics of women's self-defense training', *Violence against Women*, 20: 326–42.

CALCASA (California Coalition against Sexual Assault) (1999) *Support for Survivors: training for sexual assault counselors*. Online. Available at www.calcasa.org/wp-content/uploads/files/CALCASA-1999_Support-for-Survivors.pdf (accessed 22 December 2015).

DeGue, S., Valle, L.A., Holt, M.K., Massetti, G.M., Matjasko, J.L. and Tharp, A.T. (2014) 'A systematic review of primary prevention strategies for sexual violence perpetration', *Aggression and Violent Behavior*, 19: 346–62.

Ellsberg, M., Arango, D.J., Morton, M., Gennari, F., Kiplesund, S., Contreras, M. and Watts, C. (2015) 'Violence against women and girls 1. Prevention of violence against women and girls: what does the evidence say?' *The Lancet*, 385: 1555–66.

Gregory, D., Van Wright, S. and Wanamaker, L.M. (2015) *Self-Defense Instructor Core Competencies*. Online. Available at www.nwmaf.org/sd-instructor-core-competencies (accessed 22 December 2015).

Herman, J.L. (1997) *Trauma and Recovery: the aftermath of violence – from domestic abuse to political terror*, New York: Basic Books.

Hollander, J.A. (2014) 'Does self-defense training prevent sexual violence against women?', *Violence against Women*, 20: 252–69.

Kim, S.W., Schneider, S.M., Kravitz, L., Mermier, C. and Burge, M.R. (2013) 'Mind–body practices for posttraumatic stress disorder', *Journal of Investigative Medicine*, 61: 827–34.

LeDeux, J.E. and Gorman, J.M. (2001) 'A call to action: overcoming anxiety through active coping', *American Journal of Psychiatry*, 158: 1953–5.

McCaughey, M. and Cermele, J. (2015) 'Changing the hidden curriculum of campus rape prevention and education: women's self-defense as a key protective factor for a public health model of prevention', *Trauma, Violence and Abuse*. doi: 10.1177/1524838015611674.

Obama, B. (2014) 'Memorandum: establishing a White House Task Force to protect students from sexual assault', *Presidential Memoranda*, 22 January 2014. Online. Available at www.whitehouse.gov/the-press-office/2014/01/22/memorandum-establishing-whitehouse-task-force-protect-students-sexual-a (accessed 22 December 2015).

Rosenblum, G.D. and Taska, L.S. (2014) 'Self-defense training as clinical intervention for survivors of trauma', *Violence against Women*, 20: 293–308.

Rozee, P.D. and Koss, M.P. (2001) 'Rape: a century of resistance', *Psychology of Women Quarterly*, 25: 295–311.

Sarnquist, C., Omondi, B., Sinclair, J., Gitau, C., Paiva, L., Munyae, M., Cornfield, D.N. and Maldonado, Y. (2014) 'Rape prevention through empowerment of adolescent girls', *Pediatrics*, 133: e1226–32.

Schorn, S. (2014) 'The shark has pretty teeth, dear: why I teach women self defense', *The Hairpin*. Online. Available at http://thehairpin.com/2014/01/the-sharks-teeth/

Schorn, S. (2015) 'A look inside the terrible manual cops use to teach "rape prevention"', *Jezebel*. Online. Available at http://jezebel.com/a-look-inside-the-terrible-manual-cops-use-to-teach-rap-1687694067 (accesed 4 May 2017).

Searles, P. and Berger, R.J. (1987) 'The feminist self-defense movement: a case study', *Gender and Society*, 1: 61–84.

Senn, C.Y., Gee, S.S. and Thacke, J. (2011) 'Emancipatory sexuality education and sexual assault resistance: does the former enhance the latter?', *Psychology of Women Quarterly*, 35: 72–91.

Senn, C.Y., Eliasziw, M., Barata, P.C., Thurston, W.E., Newby-Clark, I.R., Radtke, H.L. and Hobden, K.L. (2015) 'Efficacy of a sexual assault resistance program for university women', *New England Journal of Medicine*, 372: 2326–35.

Tark, J. and Kleck, G. (2014) 'Resisting rape: the effects of victim self-protection on rape completion and injury', *Violence against Women*, 20: 270–92.

Taylor, L.R. and Wanamaker, L.M. (2014) 'How to exercise our right to defend ourselves without being victim-blaming', *Everyday Feminism*. Weblog. Available at http://everydayfeminism.com/2014/07/self-defense-blame-victims/ (accessed 18 December 2015).

Thompson, M.E. (2014) 'Empowering self-defense training', *Violence against Women*, 20: 351–9.

Trembath, S., DeFour, D., Elefante, M., Gee, J., Gorbaty, Z., Oliver, L. and Wheeler, L. (2015) *101 Skills that Will Open Doors to Effective Self-Defense Education across Cultures*. Available at www.nwmaf.org/101-ways-to-teach-across-cultures (accessed 22 December 2015).

Ullman, S.E. (2007) 'A 10-year update of "Review and critique of empirical studies of rape avoidance"', *Criminal Justice and Behavior*, 34(3): 411–29.

Ullman, S.E. (2010) *Talking about Sexual Assault: society's response to survivors*, Washington, DC: American Psychological Association. Online. Available at http://psycnet.apa.org/books/12083/ (accessed 27 June 2016).

van der Kolk, B. (2006) 'Clinical implications of neuroscience research in PTSD', *Annals of the New York Academy of Sciences*, 1071: 277–93.

van der Kolk, B., Stone, L., West, J., Rhodes, A., Emerson, D., Suvak, M. and Spinazzola, J. (2014) 'Yoga as an adjunctive treatment for posttraumatic stress disorder: a randomized controlled trial', *Journal of Clinical Psychiatry*, 75: e559–65.

WHO (2014) *Global Status Report on Violence Prevention 2014: types of violence at a glance*. Online. Available at www.who.int/violence_injury_prevention/violence/status_report/2014/report/report/en/ (accessed 22 December 2015).

8

ENGAGING BYSTANDERS IN VIOLENCE PREVENTION

Ann Taket and Cathy Plourde

Introduction

Changing social norms is a key component in achieving prevention of violence (Our Watch et al. 2015a; WHO 2010), and the potentially important role that bystanders can play has been increasingly identified (Fenton et al. 2016; Flood 2011; Our Watch et al. 2015a). This chapter explores different approaches to bystander training and the accumulating evidence on their effectiveness. It identifies the importance of engaging people in bystander work and focuses particularly on the potential of arts-based approaches for engagement, including a discussion of a theatre-based programme, *You the Man*, that is in use in the US and Australia. Findings from ongoing research in the US and Australia illustrate the value of this type of approach in diverse settings including workplaces, sporting clubs and educational institutions at both secondary and tertiary levels.

As some of the earliest work on bystanders to violence demonstrated, bystanders take action (Latané and Darley 1970) if they: notice the situation; interpret it as requiring intervention; assume responsibility; can decide what action to take; and have confidence in their skills or capacity to take action. The decades since then have seen the growth of programmes tackling the issue, but only limited research into their effectiveness. Flood (2011) concluded that there was a need for further programme development and evaluation. Since then, more research has been published, but the evidence it provides is often criticised as being weak, largely as a result of a lack of rigorous evaluation design, so that the bystander approach is often concluded to be promising, but not entirely proven (Jewkes et al. 2014). Of the most recent evidence reviews, Our Watch et al. (2015b) notes conflicting evidence, with an emphasis in many current evaluations on bystander responses to violence as opposed to its precursors; this review also notes that evaluations focus on these as stand-alone interventions rather than as a component in a wider strategy. Fenton et al. (2016), however, reviewing evidence up to 2015, concluded that positive changes from bystander interventions are evidenced across behavioural, cognitive and attitudinal measures.

Other chapters in this book have discussed programmes where bystander action is covered alongside other areas in the prevention of gender-based violence, in particular, Chapter 3 on work in schools, Chapters 4 and 5 on work with adolescents, Chapter 6 on campus-based programmes and Chapter 7 on empowerment self-defence. This chapter concentrates on programmes where the focus is on bystanders. Some of these programmes target men only, some target men and women, but are delivered separately to each group, and some are delivered to mixed groups.

In the sections below, examples of research globally on promising and proven programmes are considered first, followed by a discussion of the importance of engagement. Next the role of arts-based approaches in promoting engagement is considered, and illustrated by two case studies, one from South Africa, *Soul City*, and the second from India, *Bell Bajao!* The last major section in the chapter examines *You the Man*, looking first at its roots in the US, and then its cultural translation into Victoria, Australia.

Promising and proven programmes

In terms of specific targeted bystander programmes, *Coaching Boys into Men* is a school athletics-based programme that evaluated successfully in a cluster randomised control trial (Miller et al. 2012), provided that the programme was implemented completely. Partial implementation, involving a reduced amount of content and/ or a reduced number of weeks, produced results that were not statistically different from those in control schools. Follow-up at one year found significant reductions in dating violence perpetration (Miller et al. 2013). Das et al. (2012) report on the pilot of an India-specific cricket-based adaptation of the programme, named *Parivartan* (transformation). The evaluation of their pilot demonstrated encouraging results in terms of shifts in gender attitudes and intentions to intervene, and also reports from the female relatives of coaches and mentors about the changes they perceived in the men. *The Men's Program* (Langhinrichsen-Rohling et al. 2011) targets college men and is focused on rape prevention; the programme significantly increased self-reported willingness to help as a bystander and perceived bystander efficacy for those who attended in comparison with college men who did not. A major drawback of the study, however, was the lack of any medium- to long term follow-up. Post-intervention measures were made immediately following the programme.

The *Mentors in Violence Prevention* programme has been widely used in secondary and tertiary education, as well as the armed forces. It has been independently evaluated in high school, college, adult professional and military settings and has been proved to have positive change in participant knowledge, attitude and behaviour; some of the larger studies demonstrated statistical significance (Cissner 2009; Hollingsworth et al. 2011; Slaby et al. 2011). High school students who are exposed to the curriculum and training in the programme are more highly aware of and knowledgeable about gender violence, have less sexist or inappropriate attitudes concerning violence and harassment against women, and are more comfortable and confident in their ability to intervene in situations involving gender harassment and violence (Katz et al. 2011). Versions of the programme with different training lengths and intensities exist.

Developed for colleges and universities, the *Bringing in the Bystander®* programme was initially evaluated positively in a small study of sorority members (Moynihan et al. 2011), followed by a larger study in a mixed group (Moynihan et al. 2015) which found positive behaviour changes as long-lasting as one year following the completion of training workshops. The larger study used the longer (4.5 hours) multi-session version of the programme plus an accompanying social marketing campaign.

The University of Western England has developed the *Intervention Initiative*, provided from its website as a free resource for other universities to use (Fenton et al. 2014). This programme consists of eight sessions of 60–90 minutes, delivered by experienced facilitators. A control trial is underway, and the student achievement of learning outcomes and feedback in the latest report (Fenton and Mott 2015) is very positive.

The *Green Dot* programme (Coker et al. 2015, 2016) contains two components: 50-minute motivational speeches targeting first-year students in introductory-level courses throughout the academic year, and intensive bystander training delivered to a select group of student leaders. The training, interactive skill development, is conducted in groups of 20–25 students, lasts 4–6 hours and is provided at least once a semester. Social marketing, to staff and students, is also carried out, as well as asking faculty to endorse *Green Dot* in syllabi. The programme was implemented on one college campus and two other campuses served as comparison. Violence victimisation rates were significantly lower among students attending the campus with *Green Dot* relative to the two comparison campuses (Coker et al. 2015), and rates of sexual victimisation, sexual harassment, stalking, psychological dating violence and perpetration were all significantly lower (Coker et al. 2016).

One Act is an interpersonal violence prevention programme delivered on US college campuses (Alegría-Flores et al. 2017) developed by student leaders in collaboration with staff and faculty. The category of interpersonal violence includes sexual assault, stalking, dating violence and intimate partner violence. It is based on four hours of training, organised around a structure for positive bystander action based on four steps: observe, assess, act and follow-up. *One Act* showed significant improvements for date rape attitudes and behaviours, bystander confidence and willingness to help from pre-training to two months after training (Alegría-Flores et al. 2017). There was no statistically significant change in self-reported bystander behaviour, but note that the relatively short time before follow-up could be responsible.

Some promising bystander programmes are generic in terms of promoting citizen/community action on many issues. Many of these are rights-based programmes, educating individuals about human rights and empowering them to take action on behalf of their own and/or others' rights. As an example, Bajaj (2012) presents results from a study of the work of an Indian non-governmental organisation (NGO), the Institute of Human Rights Education, which carried out curriculum design, and then provided resources and training for teachers to deliver human rights education in government schools. The course is delivered across three years to pupils aged 11 to 15, involving two hours a week and interactive features such as stories, participatory activities and discussion questions to promote investigation into school and community realities. In later years of schooling clubs and summer camps are available. The course has been used in 18 states and more than 3,500 schools across India. The study Bajaj reports examined the impacts identified by students in interviews and focus groups. The largest reported category of impact was bystander action. So, for example, one student in a focus group reported how he and his classmates had taken action to prevent the murder of a new-born baby girl by her parents. He explained how the group of classmates visited the home and talked to the parents about their daughter's right to life. Despite receiving negative responses from the father, including scolding and slapping, the group continued to visit: 'Often we used to go to that home and watch that child. But now that child is older and is even studying in school' (Bajaj 2012: 77).

The importance of engagement

Many of the formal evaluations of the programmes mentioned above point to the difficulty of ensuring engagement or even participation (see for example Slaby et al. 2011). In some cases, programmes are delivered to 'captive' audiences, where opportunities for opting out are lessened or even absent, for example in many school settings. In other settings participation can be mandated, for example in the army (Potter and Stapleton 2012) or professional sports associations (Corboz et al. 2016), but engagement is still an issue, even if attendance is not. Arts-based approaches are suggested as one way of overcoming problems of low engagement, involving the ability of art to move people emotionally and develop an empathic understanding of the challenges faced by those who experience violence and abuse.

Arts-based approaches

As Singhal et al. (2004) describe, there is a considerable history of work that explores the use of drama of various types for different health promotion and social change purposes, arguing that suitably constructed drama can foster engagement of the participants/audience in the subject matter to positive effect. Two particular types of drama are commonly found: interactive theatre, where there is interaction between audience and actors, and education entertainment or edutainment, where media content is both entertaining and educational. While many of these programmes are aimed at health promotion topics such as HIV prevention, substance abuse, immunisation, teenage pregnancy and cancer, there are a growing number of examples that target gender-based violence in different ways.

Singhal et al. (2001) discuss the Chinese TV series *Zhonguo Baixing* (Ordinary Chinese People) which dealt with the status of girl children and women, demonstrating it raised awareness of the importance of raising gender equality, stopping harmful social and cultural practices, and boosting self- and collective efficacy. Belknap et al. (2013) describe the use of interactive theatre to address teen dating violence with Mexican American adolescents. Acceptance of teen dating violence reduced significantly after the programme, and confidence to resolve conflicts non-violently and intentions to use non-violent strategies both increased significantly. *Safe Dates*, a school-based education programme for adolescents, incorporates a theatre production performed by students and has been successfully evaluated in a randomised control trial (Foshee et al. 2004). Allen and Solomon (2016) describe the *Edutainment Violence Intervention/Prevention Model*, designed to prevent a particular form of intersectional race- and gender-based violence, specifically by working with black adolescents who have been or will be exposed to the trauma of police brutality; they report promising results. Below, examples of two well-evaluated initiatives targeted specifically at bystander engagement are considered in more detail.

Soul City, South Africa

The *Soul City* programme of work was developed by the Soul City Institute for Health and Development Communication, a South African NGO utilising mass media for social change. It involves prime time radio and television dramas and print material, and uses an edutainment approach, where social issues are integrated into entertainment formats. Through drama *Soul City* reaches prime time audiences, and through radio particularly, reaches marginalised, rural communities. Edutainment has been shown to achieve strong audience identification with characters and stories. This allows for audiences to experience the lives of the characters vicariously and is an important device to enhance feelings of individual self- and collective efficacy. The genre also allows for role modelling of positive norms, attitudes and behaviours, including help-seeking and help-giving actions. Domestic violence was a major focus of the fourth series of *Soul City*. This series aimed to impact at individual, community and socio-political levels, recognising the importance of a comprehensive multi-level approach. The development process carefully considered how best to shape the storyline and reinforced key messages about domestic violence (Usdin et al. 2004). The impact of the series was independently evaluated at individual, community, and society levels (Usdin et al. 2005). The evaluation report demonstrated that *Soul City* successfully reached 86 per cent, 65 per cent and 25 per cent of audiences through television, radio, and print booklets respectively. At the individual level there were shifts in knowledge and attitudes around domestic violence. There were also positive changes in perceptions of social norms. Qualitative data analysis suggested that *Soul City* helped enhance women's and communities' sense of efficacy. While demonstrating actual reductions in levels of domestic violence was not possible, Usdin et al. (2005) found a strong association between exposure to the various components of *Soul City* and a range of intermediary factors indicative of, and necessary for, bringing about social change. Gesser-Edelsburg and Singhal (2013) explore in some detail how the storyline in the fourth series was constructed in order to effect the desired social change.

Bell Bajao!, India

> In front of my house, there is a family that drags the woman by her hair. They drag her near the gas and say 'burn yourself'. They don't give her food. In winters I see her without warm clothes. In summers she has no fan. She stays locking [sic] a room, like a prisoner. After watching the *Bell Bajao!* ads, we started making some noise every time we heard violence. The violence used to stop for the time being. Eventually it stopped entirely. I did feel good about helping her. Earlier I used to feel helpless around her. Now she's happy, so I am happy. It was like helping my own child. I want to thank *Bell Bajao!* for inspiring me to take action.
>
> *(Quote from Indian government worker, given on Breakthrough n.d)*

Bell Bajao! ('ring the bell' in English) is a campaign aimed at prompting bystanders, particularly men and boys, to join efforts to end violence against women. An NGO, Breakthrough, has been delivering *Bell Bajao!* in India since 2008 (Silliman 2012). The strategy is based around a media campaign involving a series of television, radio and print advertisements, plus a community mobilisation initiative delivered in two states. Advertisements were disseminated widely through a partnership with the Indian Ministry of Women and Child Development. Bollywood actor Boman Irani was the campaign's first male ambassador. In the television advertisements a man or a boy hears a woman being beaten behind the closed door of her home. After a moment of deliberation, he then rings the doorbell of the woman's home. When the abuser comes to the door, the man or boy asks to borrow a cup of milk (in one advertisement) or use the phone or to retrieve a lost cricket ball (in other advertisements). It is made clear to the viewer that that the bell ringer is making the request as a pretext: he heard violence committed against the woman, and he is putting the abuser on notice that the violence will not be tolerated. The community mobilisation initiative involved leadership training, mass outreach and face-to-face educational events. Rights advocates, trained by Breakthrough in human rights and recognising and dealing with rights violations, are used within the community mobilisation initiative (Aleya 2012), acting as spokespersons and resources working with their communities and also taking up the responsibility for mobilisation activities that support the *Bell Bajao!* campaign, such as the video van. The video van includes video endorsements from local opinion leaders, and the advocates also run street theatre, puppet theatre and interactive games.

In 2010 Breakthrough released a series of three new TV advertisements asking if people had 'rung the bell' and taken action against domestic violence, featuring the stories of those who had taken action. Up to 2012, the campaign had reached more than 130 million people in India and it has won multiple awards, including the Silver Lion at the 2010 Cannes International Advertising Festival (Silliman 2012). The campaign has been subject to a range of evaluation activities, demonstrating increased knowledge and awareness about what constitutes domestic violence, increased knowledge of the Indian Protection of Women from Domestic Violence Act of 2005, changes in attitudes towards domestic violence, rising concern, and greater intervention by community members in cases of domestic violence (Aleya 2012; Chakraborty 2010). Significantly greater impacts were found in those areas with community mobilisation initiatives as well as mass media exposure (Chakraborty 2010). As Lapsansky and Chatterjee (2013) demonstrate, the campaign serves to challenge hegemonic norms, but does so in a positive non-confrontational style that offers all participants, both men and women, agency to act positively.

You the Man – engaging participants and prompting action

In this section of the chapter, the use of a theatre-based programme for bystander engagement is discussed. *You the Man* had its origins in the US, and after the two chapter authors met in 2012, they led a cultural translation of the programme for use in Victoria, Australia (Plourde et al. 2014). The subsections below explore the programme's development in the US before turning to the cultural translation into Victoria.

Roots in the US

Playwright and activist Cathy Plourde's arts and education non-profit/charity Add Verb Productions (http://addverbproductions.org) was frequently working with youth and dating violence/sexual assault groups to use theatre for either training of peer educators, or for use in peer education itself. Finding that, firstly, the disenfranchisement of males in dating violence/sexual assault prevention was high and, secondly, the intention of advocacy was not enough to avoid reinforcement of negative messages and stereotypes, she created *You the Man*, a one-man, multi-character production for use in educational settings, carefully crafting its messages and accompanying programme structure in direct consultation with trained advocates. The play was only performed by Add Verb's professional actors, and when schools or organisations booked the play, it was on condition that for each performance, local dating violence and sexual assault advocates would take part in any preparations and the post-show discussion. The programme's intention is to deliver in a dynamic, evocative format, the basic education content which these agencies would generally provide in their school- or community-based outreach, and free the advocates to engage with the audiences and individuals (Add Verb Productions n.d.). Add Verb's mission was steeped in Freirean pedagogy (Freire 1993) and Theatre of the Oppressed principles (Boal 1997), believing that the play and programme were to galvanise stakeholders, provide a platform for these agencies, and thus leave the community in a stronger position. To this end, all of the play's six male characters are bystanders, not offenders, who are confiding in the audience as they recognise violence happening around them and question how to best address it. They are honest, imperfect and evolving figures, recognisable in character as well as circumstance in nearly every type of community.

The *You the Man* programme has been in use in the US since 2002, and a longitudinal study of its impact in schools has been carried out (Plourde et al. 2016). The study examined short- and long-term impact on students' social norms, attitudes and perceptions concerning dating violence, and their intentions and behaviour when concerns of dating violence are noted. The study used pre- and post-surveys which were administered in the ninth grade (when the programme was delivered) at three schools over three years. Cohorts repeated the post-survey annually and focus groups were held two and three years after programme delivery. Plourde et al. (2016) report that many students exhibited better understanding of what constitutes dating violence, elevated perceptions of the seriousness of this issue, recognition of the importance of bystander action to prevent DV, as well as to provide critical support to individuals experiencing such harm, and increased awareness of what their options are, where to go for help, and how important it is that they do so.

Translation to Australia

In Australia, as Powell (2012) summarised, there was strong support in the general community for bystander action to address violence and discrimination against women. However, the more subtle and systemic contributors to violence against women – such as sexism and gender discrimination – are still not considered very serious or warranting of bystander action. There were also calls for programmes to encourage pro-social bystander action. Consultation with those in the field identified that although there were a number of bystander training programmes in existence, getting participants to come forward for training was a real challenge.

Presentation of findings from the US longitudinal study of *You the Man* at the American Public Health Association conference in 2012 allowed the two authors to meet and decide that it was worth investigating a cultural translation of the *You the Man* programme for use in Australia. Particularly attractive features of *You the Man* for the Victorian context were its portability and relatively low production cost. Given the length of time involved in the development and piloting of a suitable script for programmes such as this, investigation of translation rather than development anew seemed desirable.

In May 2013, a team from the Faculties of Health and Arts and Education at Deakin University, led by Ann Taket, started work on the production of an Australian version of *You the Man* in collaboration with Cathy Plourde and her team at the University of New England, Maine, US. The work started with a series of presentations on the *You the Man* programme held across Victoria. During these consultations the potential use of *You the Man* in Australia was explored. The consultations also identified a diverse range of enthusiastic individuals who wanted to be involved in the various stages of the work of producing the Australian version and piloting it across the state. The consultations confirmed that what was required was a translation of the play for the Australian cultural context rather than any extensive reworking of the play's storylines.

The Australian script for the play was produced and a series of informal readings held with a range of experts in the field of violence prevention to confirm the applicability and appropriateness of its contents. This allowed us to fine-tune the script. A highly experienced Australian director, Suzanne Chaundy, was engaged, and by the end of September two actors had been cast to join the team: Glenn Maynard and John Shearman. A third actor, Chris Asimos, joined in 2015.

Successful previews of the Australian programme were held in late 2013, and 2014 saw a pilot season in which data was collected on the short-term impact of the programme using pre- and post-surveys; this confirmed that the programme produced the same short-term impacts (4–6 weeks after delivery) as had been found in the US study. Unlike the American research, the Australian research investigated delivery in settings other than schools, namely sports clubs, workplaces, tertiary education and community venues. Feedback has been extremely positive:

> [The play and discussion] seemed to impact people on a personal level – I got the impression most could relate to either one of the characters or some of the moral dilemmas explored.

> It was fast-moving, messages were very clear, and your work on ensuring that script development supported messages in the Australian context was very apparent. The actor and director both did great jobs.

> [T]he refreshing thing about the play – no judgement and no victim blaming, the focus was on the response of family and friends to support Jana.

Short-term impact is strong: for example, 4–6 weeks after seeing *You the Man*, 80 per cent of participants (across all settings) said it had increased their sense of being able to take action on behalf of someone else. The research confirmed that the programme was equally applicable for adult audiences and a wide age range.

A comprehensive resource pack is supplied to support a local organiser in bringing *You the Man* into any local setting as a component in a wider strategy; the implementation guide in the pack is provided in five different versions for different settings: schools, tertiary education, sports clubs, workplaces and community.

Since 2014, *You the Man* has been used in a variety of different ways, for example as a part of the respectful relationships curriculum delivered in secondary schools; as a part of wider work on anti-discrimination, equity, and diversity in a university setting; connected into programmes of work on respect and responsibility in sports club settings; to launch a new equality strategy in a workplace; and in a workplace as part of activities around new provision of domestic violence leave for the workforce.

Safety and other issues

Dill-Shackleford et al. (2015) demonstrated the ability of live theatre to increase knowledge of and dispel myths about intimate partner violence. The evaluations of *You the Man* in delivery also demonstrate the ability of live theatre to increase understanding and knowledge about intimate partner violence; more than that, however, it increases participants' understanding of their potential power as a bystander. In this final section, some key issues regarding development, delivery and safety are discussed.

During the development of the programme, as Plourde et al. (2014) emphasised, the safety of participants and actor was an important consideration. Safety is one of the reasons that an interactive theatre approach was not used; other reasons are cost and increased skill requirements for the actor. Having the programme delivered into a pre-existing community rather than to a group of people who are strangers before the programme also supports safety. In all settings for programme delivery, there is a high likelihood if not certainty that victims and survivors will be in the room. In all settings there is also a high likelihood that perpetrators are also in the room. The programme sets the tone for civil/social expectation, without shame or blame. One key requirement for local organisers is to arrange for safe space and counselling resources to be provided while the programme is being delivered, so that anyone who finds the programme raises some personal issue for them can access support immediately. Should anyone leave during the play or the panel discussion, someone will follow them to check whether they are okay, or if they need to access support. These facilities are not always or even usually used during the programme; however, their existence serves to reinforce messages about support being available, and local organisers frequently report some increases in uptake of local resources after programme delivery.

The *You the Man* programme can also be seen as a rights-based approach. Dating violence, sexual assault and other forms of gender-based violence are all violations of basic human rights stemming from an abuse of power. An advantage of bystander intervention is its focus on supporting positive agency for all – demonstrating positive roles that all genders can enact, while honouring that the issues are complex. The programme demonstrates that there are steps that can be taken for positive social change.

References

Add Verb Productions (n.d.) *You the Man*. Online. Available at www.addverbproductions. org/you-the-man/ (accessed 15 March 2017).

Alegría-Flores, K., Raker, K., Pleasants, R.K., Weaver, M.A. and Weinberger, M. (2017) 'Preventing interpersonal violence on college campuses', *Journal of Interpersonal Violence*, 32: 1103–26.

Aleya, S. (2012) *Breakthrough: Bell Bajao! Campaign. Report based on stories collected for monitoring and evaluation of social change, using the most significant change technique*, New Delhi, India: Oxfam India. Online. Available at www.bellbajao.org/wp-content/uploads/2012/08/ Bell-Bajao-Most-Significant-Change-Stories1.pdf (accessed 29 March 2016).

Allen, V.D. and Solomon, P. (2016) 'EVIP-*Edutainment Violence Intervention/Prevention* model', *Journal of Human Behavior in the Social Environment*, 26: 325–35.

Bajaj, M. (2012) 'From "time pass" to transformative force: school-based human rights education in Tamil Nadu, India', *International Journal of Educational Development*, 32(1): 72–80.

Belknap, R.A., Haglund, K., Felzer, H., Pruszynski, J. and Schneider, J.A. (2013) 'Theater intervention to prevent teen dating violence for Mexican-American middle school students', *Journal of Adolescent Health*, 53: 62–7.

Boal, A. (1997) 'The theatre of the oppressed', *UNESCO Courier*, 50(11): 32–8.

Breakthrough (n.d.) *About*. Online. Available at www.bellbajao.org/home/about/ (accessed 29 March 2016).

Chakraborty, S. (2010) *End Line Survey on Domestic Violence and HIV/AIDS, 2010*. Online. Available at www.bellbajao.org/wp-content/uploads/2012/08/Bell-Bajao-Endline-Report.pdf (accessed 29 March 2016).

Cissner, A.B. (2009) *Evaluating the Mentors in Violence Prevention Programs: preventing gender violence on a college campus*, New York: Center for Court Innovation.

Coker, A.L., Fisher, B.S., Bush, H.M., Swan, S.C., Williams, C.M., Clear, E.R. and DeGue, S. (2015) 'Evaluation of the *Green Dot* bystander intervention to reduce interpersonal violence among college students across three campuses', *Violence against Women*, 21: 1507–27.

Coker, A.L., Bush, H.M., Fisher, B.S., Swan, S.C., Williams, C.M., Clear, E.R. and DeGue, S. (2016) 'Multi-college bystander intervention evaluation for violence prevention', *American Journal of Preventive Medicine*, 50: 295–302.

Corboz, J., Flood, M. and Dyson, S. (2016) 'Challenges of bystander intervention in male-dominated professional sport: lessons from the Australian Football League', *Violence against Women*, 22: 324–43.

Das, M., Ghosh, S., Miller, E., O'Conner, B. and Verma, R. (2012) *Engaging Coaches and Athletes in Fostering Gender Equity: findings from the Parivartan program in Mumbai, India*, New Delhi: ICRW and Futures Without Violence.

Dill-Shackleford, K.E., Green, M.C., Scharrer, E., Wetterer, C. and Shackleford, L.E. (2015) 'Setting the stage for social change: using live theater to dispel myths about intimate partner violence', *Journal of Health Communication*, 20: 969–76.

Fenton, R.A. and Mott, H.L. (2015) *The Intervention Initiative: student feedback February 2015*, Bristol: University of the West of England. Online. Available at https://public.uwe.ac.uk/ faculties/BBS/BUS/law/Law%20docs/bystander/Partners/Student_Feedback_report. pdf (accessed 7 March 2017).

Fenton, R.A., Mott, H.L., McCartan, K. and Rumney, P.N.S. (2014) *The Intervention Initiative*, Bristol: University of the West of England and Public Health England. Online. Available at www.uwe.ac.uk/bl/research/InterventionInitiative (accessed 3 May 2016).

Fenton, R.A., Mott, H.L., McCartan, K. and Rumney, P.N.S. (2016) *A Review of Evidence for Bystander Intervention to Prevent Sexual and Domestic Violence in Universities*, London: Public Health England.

Flood, M. (2011) 'Involving men in efforts to end violence against women and children', *Men and Masculinities*, 14(3): 358–77.

Foshee V.A., Bauman, K.E., Ennett, S.T., Linder, G.F., Benefield, T. and Suchindran, C. (2004) 'Assessing the long-term effects of the *Safe Dates* program and a booster in preventing and reducing adolescent dating violence victimization and perpetration', *American Journal of Public Health*, 94: 619–24.

Freire, P. (1993) *Pedagogy of the Oppressed*, new revised 20th anniversary edition, New York: Continuum.

Gesser-Edelsburg, A. and Singhal, A. (2013) 'Enhancing the persuasive influence of entertainment-education events: rhetorical and aesthetic strategies for constructing narratives', *Critical Arts-South-North Cultural and Media Studies*, 27: 56–74.

Hollingsworth, C., Ramsey, K.J. and Hadley, J.A. (2011) *Bystander Intervention Pilot: final report*, Virginia Beach, VA: Department of the Navy.

Jewkes, R., Flood, M. and Lang, J. (2014) 'From work with men and boys to changes of social norms and reduction of inequities in gender relations: a conceptual shift in prevention of violence against women and girls', *Lancet* 385: 1580–9.

Katz, J., Heisterkamp, H.A. and Fleming, W.M. (2011) 'The social justice roots of the *Mentors in Violence Prevention* model and its application in a high school setting', *Violence against Women*, 17: 684–702.

Langhinrichsen-Rohling, J., Foubert, J.D., Brasfield, H.M., Hill, B. and Shelley-Tremblay, S. (2011) '*The Men's Program*: does it impact college men's self-reported bystander efficacy and willingness to intervene?' *Violence against Women*, 17(6): 743–59.

Lapsansky, C., and Chatterjee, J. (2013) 'Masculinity matters: using entertainment education to engage men in ending violence in India', *Critical Arts*, 27(1): 36–55.

Latané, B. and Darley, J. (1970) *The Unresponsive Bystander: why doesn't he help?* New York: Appleton-Century-Crofts.

Miller, E., Tancredi, D.J., McCauley, H.L., Decker, M.R., Virata, M.C.D., Anderson, H.A., Stetkevich, N., Brown, E.W., Moideen, F. and Silverman, J.G. (2012) '*Coaching Boys into Men*: a cluster-randomized controlled trial of a dating violence prevention program', *Journal of Adolescent Health*, 51(5): 431–8.

Miller, E., Tancredi, D.J., MacCauley, H.L., Decker, M.R., Virata, M.D., Anderson, H.A., O'Connor, B. and Silverman, J.G. (2013) 'One-year follow-up of a coach-delivered dating violence prevention program: a clustered randomized controlled trial', *American Journal of Preventive Medicine*, 45(1): 108–12.

Moynihan, M.M., Banyard, V.L., Arnold, J.S., Eckstein, R.P. and Stapleton, J.G. (2011) 'Sisterhood may be powerful for reducing sexual and intimate partner violence: an evaluation of the *Bringing in the Bystander* in-person program with sorority members', *Violence against Women*, 17: 703–19.

Moynihan, M.M., Banyard, V.L., Cares, A.C., Potter, S.J., Williams, L.M. and Stapleton, J.G. (2015) 'Encouraging responses in sexual and relationship violence prevention: what program effects remain 1 year later?', *Journal of Interpersonal Violence*, 30: 110–32.

Our Watch, Australia's National Research Organisation for Women's Safety, and Victorian Health Promotion Foundation (2015a) *Change the Story: a shared framework for the primary prevention of violence against women and their children in Australia*. Melbourne: Our Watch.

Our Watch, Australia's National Research Organisation for Women's Safety, and VicHealth (2015b) *Framework Foundations 1: a review of the evidence on correlates of violence against women and what works to prevent it. Companion document to Change the Story: a shared framework for the primary prevention of violence against women and their children in Australia.* Melbourne: Our Watch.

Plourde, C., Taket, A., Murray, V. and van der Werf, P. (2014) 'The development and cultural translation of a brief theatre-based program for the promotion of bystander engagement and violence prevention', *Journal of Applied Arts and Health*, 5(3): 377–92.

Plourde, C., Shore, N., Herrick, P., Morrill, A., Cattabriga, G., Bottino, L., Orme, E. and Stromgren, C. (2016) '*You the Man*: theater as bystander education in dating violence', *Arts and Health*, 8: 229–47.

Potter, S.J. and Stapleton, J.G. (2012) 'Translating sexual assault prevention from a college campus to a United States military installation: piloting the *Know-Your-Power* bystander social marketing campaign', *Journal of Interpersonal Violence*, 27: 1593–621.

Powell, A. (2012) *More than Ready: bystander action to prevent violence against women in the Victorian community*, Melbourne: VicHealth research report.

Silliman, J. (2012) '*Bell Bajao!* as a case study', in *Communications and Technology for Violence Prevention: proceedings of a workshop*, Washington, DC: National Academies Press.

Singhal, A., Vaughan, P., Ren, L. and Zhang, J. (2001) *Impact of Zhongguo Baixing, an Entertainment Education Television Series, on Gender Equity and Family Planning in China*, Beijing: Ford Foundation.

Singhal, A., Cody, M.J., Rogers, E. and Sabido, M. (eds) (2004) *Entertainment Education and Social Change: history, research and practice*, Mahwah, NJ: Lawrence Erlbaum Associates.

Slaby, R., Branner, A. and Martin, S. (2011) *Mentors in Violence Prevention: an evaluation of the 2009–2011 Campus Leadership Initiative Program*, Washington, DC: US Department of Justice Office on Violence against Women.

Usdin, S., Singhal, A., Shongwe, T., Goldstein, S., and Shabalala, A. (2004) 'No short cuts in entertainment education: designing *Soul City* step by step', in A. Singhal, M. J. Cody, E. Rogers and M. Sabido (eds) *Entertainment Education and Social Change: history, research and practice*, Mahwah, NJ: Lawrence Erlbaum Associates.

Usdin, S., Scheepers, E., Goldstein, S. and Japhet, G. (2005) 'Achieving social change on gender-based violence: a report on the impact evaluation of *Soul City*'s fourth series', *Social Science and Medicine*, 61(11), 2434–45.

WHO (2010) *Preventing Intimate Partner Violence and Sexual Violence against Women: taking action and generating evidence*, Geneva: World Health Organization.

9

FAITH COMMUNITIES AS A SETTING FOR THE PREVENTION OF GENDER-BASED VIOLENCE

Beth R. Crisp

Introduction

Five out of every six people (84 per cent) living on earth report identifying with one of the world's religions (Pew Research Center 2012). While the numbers of those who regularly participate in activities associated with religious institutions are far fewer than those who identify with religions (Crisp 2013), the reach of religious groups is nevertheless considerable and often extends far beyond that of other services (Strickland et al. 1998). However, many health and welfare professionals have been unable to grasp the potential of working with faith-based organisations on health promotion programmes generally (Ayton et al. 2012). Hence, this chapter explores the ways in which religious organisations can play a role in preventing gender-based violence (GBV), and the issues that may emerge with such initiatives.

One of the obstacles to recognising the potential of faith-based initiatives in the prevention of gender-based violence is that certain perceptions of reality are often regarded as universal truths, despite considerable evidence to the contrary. In particular, careful consideration of the following myths is required:

1. Gender-based violence does not occur in religious communities.
2. Religious communities are not interested in tackling gender-based violence.
3. Gender-based violence is supported by religious beliefs.
4. Religious communities are not an appropriate place to challenge gender-based violence.

Each of these myths will be discussed in turn, before introducing some initiatives which illustrate that faith-based organisations can play a role in the prevention of gender-based violence. While acknowledging that GBV is not aligned with any one religious tradition (Dorff 2014; Grey 2010), this chapter will predominantly focus on responses to this problem within Christianity.

Dispelling myths

Myth 1: Gender-based violence does not occur in religious communities

Arguably, the first requirement of any community in responding to gender-based violence is recognition that this is an issue within the community. Indeed, it is not unheard of for religious leaders to deny that GBV occurs within their communities (Horsburgh 1995). Alternatively, some church leaders will acknowledge its existence, but minimise the impact by stating that it occurs much less frequently in their faith communities than in the wider society (Horne and Levitt 2003). Consequently, it is rare for churches to promote information about GBV and services established to tackle this societal problem (Manetta et al. 2003). Nevertheless, a lack of public recognition can occur despite GBV having been entrenched in the culture for hundreds or even thousands of years (Cwik 1995).

While the responses of church leaders who deny the presence of GBV may be naïve, a culture of silence within the religious community may at the same time have resulted in leaders having no evidence to support the notion that it is present in their communities (Dyer 2010). Hence, even if they do not mean to do so, members of a church community can be complicit in keeping the problem of GBV concealed (Knickmeyer et al. 2010). Therefore, church leaders may need to break any code of silence which prevents discussion about GBV within their communities:

> Once named and no longer invisible, sexual violence moves from the margin to the center of a discussion about women's lives. For the church to be effective, this movement of the issue of sexual violence from margin to center must occur within its own structures.
>
> Church leaders must acknowledge that they *know* sexual violence exists in society, and, therefore, in their congregations. Are they prepared to offer helpful responses? When clergy *do* name violence from the pulpit or in their other capacities as church leaders, they report surprise at the number of people who come forward who have personally been affected by sexual violence.
>
> *(Adams 1993: 62)*

Others have also reported that on becoming aware of gender-based violence within religious communities, leaders have not only responded to individual situations but have spoken out about the issue within the community (Dyer 2010; Horsburgh 1995). The problem of a lack of awareness will be addressed later in this chapter in an exploration of awareness-raising actions undertaken by the World Council of Churches.

Myth 2: Religious communities are not interested in tackling gender-based violence

One interpretation of the lack of response to the issue is that religious communities are not interested in tackling it. Undoubtedly, there are contexts in which this is the reality. However, an awareness of the issues does not necessarily translate into knowing *how* to respond appropriately to either specific instances of gender-based violence or the issue of GBV more generally (Knickmeyer et al. 2010; Wendt 2008). Indeed, there may be considerable awareness of GBV occurring within a community and a recognition that mishandling the problem may actually make things worse for vulnerable members (Mitchell 2012).

Religious communities may in fact need support and encouragement if they are to start tackling issues associated with GBV. In particular, they may fail to realise how their teachings could be a resource in promoting non-violent relationships (Wendt 2008). Nuancing, however, is important, as a well-intended intervention could have an effect opposite to that which was intended, particularly in respect of actions by clergy. For example, it has been suggested that

> ministers have a tendency to minimize the lethality of sexual and domestic violence by focusing instead on relationship issues. This distorts the responsibility of the abuser . . . [I]nadequate counseling techniques are taken as adequate . . . When untrained to identify and act on the evidence of sexual and domestic violence, ministers will put women at risk if they follow traditional counseling techniques.
>
> *(Adams 1993: 67)*

Clearly if they are to be effective in responding to GBV, religious leaders need training around domestic violence (Wendt 2008). Furthermore, thanks to both the influence they have within their communities and the reach they have into the lives of their members, religious leaders are starting to be considered in efforts to prevent GBV (Colpitts 2014). Some approaches to this are taken up later in this chapter in the section on developing capacity among church leaders to tackle gender-based violence.

Myth 3: Gender-based violence is supported by religious beliefs

In addition to myths which propose that religious communities are not interested in addressing gender-based violence, religious texts and other teachings have often been interpreted as condoning it (Grey 2010; Messina-Dysert 2015). However, in what have been labelled 'cultural distortions' of religion (Ayyub 2000: 247), the original intent of texts may have been distorted. For example, a study of female Muslim survivors of abuse found that some interpreted a Koranic text about not hitting someone on the face and head and ensuring that hitting does not leave a mark as being protective of them, whereas others found the same text oppressive (Hassouneh-Phillips 2003). Even so, many Muslims deny that the Koran allows for gendered violence, and would argue that their religion argues for the protection of vulnerable members of the community (Hussain 2012).

Contradictory interpretations of texts have also occurred in Christianity such that Isherwood (2003: 212) has written that 'a dangerous connection is made between the abuse of women and the working out of God's purpose'. In traditions in which the maleness of God is emphasised, women are not necessarily considered to be properly *Imago Dei* (in the image of God), and are treated with less reverence (Clavero White et al. 2010). And it is perhaps unsurprising that a theology which emphasises the fallenness of all women since Eve may fail to recognise the existence of gender-based violence or promote equality between men and women (West 1999). Furthermore, the othering of women, particularly in respect of a male God, has legitimated GBV in some religious traditions (Hunt 1996).

Women who grew up in religious families where GBV was sanctioned may have had reduced ability to avoid violence in their own marriages as a result of not being able to recognise signs of abuse such as controlling behaviours early in a relationship (Giesbrecht and Sevcik 2000). Similarly, even if they did not experience violence in their families of origin, women who grew up in families who lived according to religious teachings in which the gender norms were of female compliance and passivity may have difficulties protecting themselves and any children from violence in the home (Levitt and Ware 2006), particularly if religious teachings also proscribe divorce and encourage victims to blame themselves (Giesbrecht and Sevcik 2000):

> the salubrious dynamics of the family unit is regarded as one of the founda-
> tional components of a moral and spiritual life. For this purpose, the alliance
> between a husband and a wife . . . [has] been decreed with much detail in a
> variety of religious texts.
>
> *(Rahim 2000: 188)*

If religious women are disempowered from taking action to protect themselves against violence, they may also be disadvantaged by a culture which inhibits bystanders, such as members of the extended family, from advocating for them or offering protection to women (Ayyub 2000). Moreover, if they are given assistance, women may be offered therapy rather than being assisted to tackle systemic issues which have contributed to them being subjected to violence (West 1999).

Despite religious beliefs and practices having a long history of inciting violence, it can be forgotten that they also have a tradition of promoting peace and non-violence (Mitchell 2012). However, realising cultural change within churches is difficult to achieve without the active involvement of theologians (McMullen 2003). As the British theologian Mary Grey explains,

> Resisting violence is a deeply spiritual work . . . We must deconstruct theolo-
> gies of the spirit that devalue physical life, especially life as symbolized in the
> bodies, and particularly the sexuality, of women. Spirit/body dualism must be

reconstructed toward a whole life energy of resisting, renewing, sustaining, healing, and growing.

(Grey 1996: 52)

Nevertheless, paternalistic beliefs of male clergy continue to 'endanger' many women (Jacinto et al. 2010: 112) and the inadequacy of much theological education in preparing clergy to respond to gender-based violence in their work is long recognised (Adams 1993). Hence, an example of the provision of theological education which seeks to confront rather than reinforce GBV is a strategy for violence prevention which will be discussed later in this chapter.

Myth 4: Religious communities are not an appropriate place to challenge gender-based violence

As expectations about violence and abuse are influenced by the social context (Chiswell 2012), community members may regard the church as having the power to set precedents around responding to domestic violence (Knickmeyer et al. 2010; Wendt 2008). Indeed,

> The Churches have for generations spoken up for victims of torture under political regimes around the world. The reality is that the violence that many women suffer is as brutal and psychologically more devastating since a loved one carries it out, but the Churches have, until very recently, remained silent.
>
> *(Isherwood 2003: 205)*

Consequently,

> When it fails to help the victim, it [the church] simultaneously colludes with the rapist while demonstrating its powerlessness to him. The rapist is thus enabled to view the church and its representatives with the same scorn he holds for his victim. And the victim faces further violence, deserted by her faith community and, from her perspective, by her God as well.
>
> *(Adams 1993: 59–60)*

Thanks to the respect they command within, and even beyond, their communities, religious leaders can be influential in setting community standards concerning 'not only what is considered acceptable within the family unit, but the response to unacceptable behavior as well' (Shannon-Lewy and Dull 2005: 649). Therefore,

> Both women and men are able to make significant changes when they begin to recognize the limitations of traditional femininities and masculinities and explore new subjectivities that confront issues of power and control in personal relationships. The church can play a major role by exploring these new subjectivities.
>
> *(Wendt 2008: 152)*

Furthermore, it has been argued that religious leaders who are not proactive in speaking out publicly against gender-based violence are unlikely to be perceived as credible sources of support by women who have experienced abuse (Burnett 1996). As clergy also frequently fulfil the role of gatekeepers to community services, both those provided by their churches and also other services (Dyer 2010), their willingness or not to refer women to specialist support services is also critical in letting it be known what is considered acceptable behaviour within the community.

Strategies which respond to these myths

This section provides examples of initiatives which explicitly challenge common myths about gender-based violence in religious communities.

Strategy 1: Developing awareness – World Council of Churches

The myth that gender-based violence does not occur in religious communities has been challenged at an international level by various initiatives of the World Council of Churches (WCC), which is the largest peak organisation of Christian churches, representing 500 million members (WCC 2016). The years 1988–98 were designated by the WCC as the Ecumenical Decade of Churches in Solidarity with Women. Member churches, nationally and locally, were encouraged to create spaces for the wider church to enable 'women to share their spirituality, their daily struggles and their gifts' (Kessler 1999: 243). One of the key issues which emerged over this decade was calls from women for churches to stand in solidarity with women who experienced gender-based violence. Questions being asked by women of their churches included:

> Has the Christian church openly discussed and addressed gender violence as a justice issue? Have we named it in our prayers? Do we preach about the dignity and worth of women, and against the sin of abuse? Have we publicly acknowledged our historical complicity? Have we campaigned for the political and legal changes required to ensure female equality and safety? . . . How many wounded people experience the church as a secure, holding yet invigorating environment, which offers us all the space to flourish? How can we be a place of God's presence – a sanctuary – if we do not honour the sacredness of God in the bodies and spirits of those who suffer abuse?
>
> *(Orr Macdonald 2000: 33)*

The achievements of the Ecumenical Decade of Churches in Solidarity with Women were reviewed at a conference in Harare in November 1998, which was attended by more than one thousand women and approximately thirty men (Kessler 1999). Many participants spoke about different forms of violence in the church and called for churches to both acknowledge this violence and seek to change the culture of violence both in the churches and in broader society.

While opening up discussion and identifying how widespread abuse is in church communities was an important first step, participants at the Harare conference also developed a set of recommendations for actions. These were presented to the subsequent WCC meetings, also held in Harare in 1998. Consequently, the WCC's next major response was to designate the years from 2001 to 2010 to be the Decade to Overcome Violence (DOV). While not specifically focusing on gender-based violence, some of the activities did have this focus.

At a consultation in Dundee in 2001 to mark the beginning of the Decade to Overcome Violence participants spoke of a range of initiatives already occurring. These included support being offered by local churches to women experiencing domestic violence or sexual abuse, gender awareness training being included in the education of clergy, and policies and procedures designed to prevent and respond to gender-based violence in religious institutions. Nevertheless, they recognised that there was still much which needed doing and proposed a set of *General Principles and Objectives to Overcome All Forms of Violence against Women* to 'adopt an agenda which will address all issues that concern violence against women and its consequences for individuals, faith communities and societies' (Hood 2003: 225). This included recognition of the need for theological reflection, education within church communities, development of safe environments in which violence is not tolerated and working in partnership with other community organisations seeking to prevent violence.

The work of the DOV largely happened in national and local churches around the world. Over the decade, many resources were developed and made available internationally. The final report includes many examples of 'Good Practice' in different regions, which can be adapted within local settings. The WCC's evaluation of the DOV recognised that while much had been achieved, there were still many challenges in overcoming violence both generally, and particularly in respect of violence against women:

> It is difficult to measure the Decade's achievements in programmatic terms. However, the endeavours of so many individuals and organizations over a period of ten years have contributed to an essential shift in ways that will last. The DOV increased the churches' awareness that peace is a gift of God and offered more differentiated analyses of peace than many churches had known previously. The DOV was a beginning. It is up to us all to continue the work.
> *(WCC 2011: 133)*

Strategy 2: Developing capacity among church leaders to tackle gender-based violence – the South African Faith and Family Institute

The South African Faith and Family Institute (SAFFI) was founded in 2010 by Elizabeth Petersen, a Christian social worker in the Western Cape Region. After graduation she worked as a social worker in a shelter for abused women and came to realise the need for efforts to prevent the violence being experienced by the women she was working with rather than waiting until violence had occurred and providing services then. While many of the women were religious, their experiences of faith communities had generally been that of being told to be submissive. Elizabeth realised that making a difference would require engaging with religious leaders and, on receiving encouragement from some individuals who understood her vision, she established SAFFI as an interfaith initiative to challenge abuse within religious communities (Petersen 2013).

SAFFI now has staff and board members from a range of religious backgrounds including Christianity, Judaism, Islam and Hinduism. In addition to working with leaders in these faith communities, it has also engaged with other faith communities including Bahai. In particular, SAFFI considers its mission as:

> To advance a coordinated, multi-sectoral, culturally competent restorative justice response to violence against women and children by:
>
> * Being a resource to religious leaders, institutions and faith communities as they hold offenders accountable and ensure the safety and empowerment of victims/survivors by offering opportunity for truth telling and healing of individuals and families.
> * To challenge, from a theological perspective, patriarchal traditions and other root causes of intimate partner abuse and violence that destroys the dignity of women, children and men, and
> * To encourage the promotion of scriptural and the theological teachings that encourage intimate relationships that set people free to live their full potential in supportive unions.
>
> *(SAFFI 2014a: inner front cover)*

Training and capacity-building of religious leaders is a key aspect of the work. In 2013–14, SAFFI training programmes made contact with 185 religious leaders. While the majority of these attended half-day workshops, 60 participated in five-day training events:

> many religious leaders report an increased awareness and sensitivity when it comes to their preaching. Many report that they now are able to identify signs of domestic violence during pastoral care of couples who present with marital problems. One pastor said, 'now I understand what feminists have been trying to tell us for years about the link between patriarchy and intimate partner abuse. I can now see clearly see how my preaching can make an enormous difference.'
>
> *(SAFFI 2014a: 7)*

While the extent of published evaluations seems to be positive from comments from participants included in annual reports and other publicity, an important strength of SAFFI is being able to be reflective as to what is working and adopt new approaches if these seem more promising (SAFFI 2014a).

In addition to providing education to religious leaders, SAFFI has also been involved in education and advocacy more broadly in the Western Cape community through having a media presence and developing partnerships with other organisations (SAFFI 2014a). In December 2014 it established a Theological Advisory Council on Gender-Based Violence which at its inception involved 18 scholars and leaders from various religious traditions who pledged their commitment to challenging theological misconceptions which result when religious teachings are misinterpreted so as to sanction or not proscribe gender-based violence. The Theological Advisory Council anticipates acting as a resource to different faith traditions around the development of policies, procedures and resources for the prevention of GBV which have theological integrity for a faith community, as well as being a resource to other GBV service providers in respect of religious issues (SAFFI 2014b).

Strategy 3: Transforming theological education – Pacific Theological College, Fiji

Whereas organisations like SAFFI are primarily working with existing leaders, another important strategy is to ensure that new generations of religious leaders are trained to prevent, rather than perpetuate and/or even perpetrate, gender-based violence in their communities. In particular, it has been recognised that they may need opportunities to explore perceived contradictions between their religious beliefs and societal expectations concerning gender roles (Shannon-Lewy and Dull 2005).

Recognising the need to include issues of gender and violence in the theological curriculum, Joan Alleluia Filemoni-Tofaeono and Lydia Johnson, who were teaching at the Pacific Theological College in Fiji, began this process by introducing a year-long programme for final-year students, most of whom were training for the ministry in churches in the Oceania region. Part of their rationale was as follows:

> The silence of many churches on the issue of violence against women, particularly its more subtle forms such as harassment, is thus a reflection of ecclesial complicity in the perpetuation of patriarchal theology. The church's silence has contributed to the invisibility of Christian women's suffering from male abuse . . . Clearly the church will be unable to break through its silence on or acquiescence in violence against women until it has grappled with its larger embrace of patriarchal models of leadership which have marginalized and disempowered women, and thus made them more vulnerable to abuse.
>
> *(Filemoni-Tofaeono and Johnson 2006: 106)*

Ultimately, they recognised that is was not enough just to ensure the curriculum included discussion of gender issues. Theological institutions in the region not only frequently gave the impression that violence against children, parishioners and spouses was tolerated, but may well have encouraged such behaviour by failing to challenge violence within the institution. Hence, cultural change within the theological college was essential, although difficult to achieve if not supported by the broader church community (Filemoni-Tofaeono and Johnson 2006).

Strategy 4: Developing denominational policies – the Anglican Diocese of Melbourne

In 1989 the Evangelical Lutheran Church in America developed a policy to make the church a safe place where sexual harassment and sexual abuse would not be tolerated and resolved that the church would work to eliminate such practices (Cooper-White 1995). By the mid-1990s, guidance as to what church policies concerning gender-based violence should include was emerging, although most tended to be more concerned with responding to incidents of abuse than prevention (Cooper-White 1995; Fortune and Poling 1995). Furthermore, key considerations in the development of denominational policies in the 1980s and 1990s were frequently financial and the fear of being sued for not having adequate policies and procedures (Timmerman 1993), rather than recognising the prevention of GBV as a human rights issue (Amenga-Etego 2006).

Rather than continue the focus primarily on reactive approaches, a preventive approach to violence against women has been adopted by the synod of the Anglican Diocese of Melbourne. In 2011, the synod meetings adopted a policy which sought to promote respectful relationships both at the diocesan level and filtering down to local parishes. Importantly, the proposal was endorsed by the archdiocese's Social Responsibilities Commission which has the mandate to bring social justice matters to the notice of the synod. Furthermore, the chair of this committee, who became the public spokesperson for the work which ensued from the adoption of the policy, was a bishop, i.e. one of the most senior ranking clergy in the diocese (Holmes 2012).

On accepting the policy, funds were provided for the appointment of a project worker to coordinate the policy implementation. Activities in the first two years included research, running training sessions for clergy and theological students, peer mentoring for parish leaders planning on implementing prevention of violence against women programmes in their local churches, development of resources to be used in parish and wider church contexts, a social media presence and development of materials for inclusion in church media (Boddé 2013, 2014). Evaluations indicate impressive progress when taking into account the very limited hours for which the programme coordinator was employed, but also that much work is still needed to overcome the structural and cultural inequalities associated with violence against women, and to strengthen what works to prevent it (Boddé 2013).

Conclusion

Preventing, rather than responding to, gender-based violence is a relatively new concept for many faith-based communities. Nevertheless, suggestions that religious communities are not open to addressing issues of GBV are not only untrue in many instances, but may actually hinder opportunities to engage with churches about violence. Even churches which are known to be theologically very conservative have been active participants in programmes challenging GBV (City of Casey 2009).

Initiatives which seem particularly promising are those that engage with the religious beliefs of potential perpetrators of GBV. As the report of one Australian initiative concluded:

> The findings suggest that there continue to be both challenges and opportunities for capacity building for primary prevention within the faith setting. Challenges include those generated by the patriarchal paradigms of many faith traditions, the need to develop advocates and mechanisms for capacity building, and the complexity of addressing gender issues in an interfaith context. Opportunities include the value of peer based capacity building programs, the potential for faith specific programs, resources and policy development, and the growing commitment of the faith sector to preventing violence against women.
>
> *(Holmes 2012: 7)*

However, evaluation has often been limited. Specific project reports are produced as a requirement when there has been external funding, but this tends to only be for evaluating initial impacts or activities rather than longer-term outcomes (Holmes 2012). For initiatives which have been funded within the religious community, there may be no requirement for the work to be formally evaluated. Evaluation is important as well-intentioned initiatives can have an effect very different from that which was anticipated:

> the Church could be seen as participating – intentionally or unintentionally – in keeping and perpetuating further, some of the traditional discriminatory and violent practices against women . . . since the aspects dealing with the male members of society are not addressed and they are conveniently given an alibi in the devil.
>
> *(Amenga-Etego 2006: 39)*

Notwithstanding the difficulties which may emerge, community initiatives that seek to prevent violence against women may have much to gain by partnering with faith-based communities (Holmes 2012). Such collaborations may also benefit religious communities, as those who respond appropriately to gender-based violence are more likely to retain members when it occurs (Gillum et al. 2006). However, secular and religious partners will need to work together as initiatives which do not address the cultural and theological issues associated with gender-based violence in religious communities will be less than effective (Ayton et al. 2012).

References

Adams, C.J. (1993) '"I just raped my wife! What are you going to do about it, Pastor?" The church and sexual violence', in E. Buchwald, P.R. Fletcher and M. Roth (eds) *Transforming a Rape Culture*, Minneapolis: Milkweed Editions.

Amenga-Etego, R.M. (2006) 'Violence against women in contemporary Ghanaian society', *Theology and Sexuality*, 13(1): 23–46.

Ayton, D., Carey, G., Keleher, H. and Smith, B. (2012) 'Historical overview of church involvement in health and wellbeing in Australia: implications for health promotion partnerships', *Australian Journal of Primary Health*, 18(1): 4–10.

Ayyub, R. (2000) 'Domestic violence in the South Asian Muslim immigrant population in the United States', *Journal of Social Distress and the Homeless*, 9(3): 237–48.

Boddé, R. (2013) *Preventing Violence against Women: what works and what doesn't in Anglican communities*, Melbourne: Anglican Diocese of Melbourne. Online. Available at www.anglican. org.au/home/documents/news-and-media-releases/preventing%20violence%20 against%20women%20%282013%29.pdf (accessed 15 January 2016).

Boddé, R. (2014) *Nudging Anglican Parishes to Prevent Violence against Women*, Melbourne: Anglican Diocese of Melbourne. Online. Available at http://repository.divinity.edu. au/1400/ (accessed 15 January 2016).

Burnett, M.N. (1996) 'Suffering and sanctification: the religious context of battered women's syndrome', *Pastoral Psychology*, 44(3): 145–9.

Chiswell, M. (2012) 'Addressing the sexual and reproductive health needs of adolescents in South Africa', in A. Taket (ed.) *Health Equity, Social Justice and Human Rights*, London: Routledge.

City of Casey (2009) *Promoting Peace in Families Model Package*. Online. Available at www. casey.vic.gov.au/health-safety/health-promotion/family-violence-prevention (accessed 15 January 2016).

Clavero White, C., Solares, M., Starr, R. and Ukaski, M.C. (2010) 'Violence against women in the River Plate Region: networks of resistance', *Feminist Theology*, 18(3): 294–308.

Colpitts, E. (2014) 'Working with men to prevent and address violence against women: South African perspectives', Master of Arts thesis, Dalhousie University, Canada. Online. Available at http://dalspace.library.dal.ca/handle/10222/53993 (accessed 20 March 2015).

Cooper-White, P. (1995) *The Cry of Tamar: violence against women and the church's response*, Minneapolis: Fortress Press.

Crisp, B.R. (2013) 'Social work and faith-based agencies in Sweden and Australia', *International Social Work*, 56(3): 343–55.

Cwik, M.S. (1995) 'Couples at risk? A feminist exploration of why spousal abuse may develop within Orthodox Jewish marriages', *Family Therapy*, 22(3): 165–83.

Dorff, E.N. (2014) 'Jewish provisions for protecting children', *Child Abuse and Neglect*, 38(4): 567–75.

Dyer, J. (2010) 'Challenging assumptions: clergy perspectives and practices regarding intimate partner violence', *Journal of Religion and Spirituality in Social Work*, 29(1): 33–48.

Filemoni-Tofaeono, J.A. and Johnson, L. (2006) *Reweaving the Relational Mat: a Christian response to violence against women from Oceania*, London: Equinox.

Fortune, M.M. and Poling, J. (1995) 'Calling to accountability: the church's response to abusers', in C.J. Adams and M.M. Fortune (eds) *Violence against women and children: a Christian theological sourcebook*, New York: Continuum.

Giesbrecht, N. and Sevcik, I. (2000) 'The process of recovery and rebuilding among abused women in the conservative evangelical subculture', *Journal of Family Violence*, 15(3): 229–48.

Gillum, T.L., Sullivan, C.M. and Bybee, D.I. (2006) 'The importance of spirituality in the lives of domestic violence survivors', *Violence against Women*, 12(3): 240–50.

Grey, M. (1996) 'Final statement of the "Women against Violence" dialogues', *Feminist Theology*, 4: 46–54.

Grey, M.C. (2010) *A Cry for Dignity: religion, violence and the struggle of Dalit women in India*, London: Equinox.

Hassouneh-Phillips, D. (2003) 'Strength and vulnerability: spirituality in abused American Muslim women's lives', *Issues in Mental Health Nursing*, 24(6–7): 681–94.

Holmes, S. (2012) *Northern Interfaith Respectful Relationships: project report*. Online. Available at www.vichealth.vic.gov.au/~/media/ResourceCentre/PublicationsandResources/ PVAW/Sharing%20the%20evidence_NIRR%202012.pdf?la=en (accessed 15 January 2016).

Hood, H. (2003) 'Speaking out and doing justice: it's no longer a secret but what are the churches doing about overcoming violence against women?', *Feminist Theology*, 11(2): 216–25.

Horne, S.G. and Levitt, H.M. (2003) 'Shelter from the raging wind: religious needs of victims of intimate partner violence and faith leader responses', *Journal of Religion and Abuse*, 5(2): 83–97.

Horsburgh, B. (1995) 'Lifting the veil of secrecy: domestic violence in the Jewish community', *Harvard Women's Law Journal*, 18: 171–217.

Hunt, M.E. (1996) 'Change or be changed: Roman Catholicism and violence', *Feminist Theology*, 4: 43–60.

Hussain, M. (2012) 'Islam and the news', in J. Mitchell and O. Gower (eds) *Religion and the News*, Farnham: Ashgate.

Isherwood, L. (2003) 'Marriage: haven or hell? Twin souls and broken bones', *Feminist Theology*, 11(2): 203–15.

Jacinto, G.A., Turnage, B.F. and Cook, I. (2010) 'Domestic violence survivors: spirituality and social support', *Journal of Religion and Spirituality in Social Work*, 29(2): 109–23.

Kessler, D. (ed.) (1999) *Together on the Way: official report of the eighth assembly of the World Council of Churches*, Geneva: World Council of Churches.

Knickmeyer, N., Levitt, H. and Horne, S.G. (2010) 'Putting on Sunday best: the silencing of battered women within Christian faith communities', *Feminism and Psychology*, 20(1): 94–113.

Levitt, H.M. and Ware, K.G. (2006) '"Anything with two heads is a monster": religious leaders' perspectives on marital equality and domestic violence', *Violence against Women*, 12(12): 1169–90.

McMullen, C. (2003) 'One day I went to a theological consultation on domestic violence', *Feminist Theology*, 11(2): 197–202.

Manetta, A.A., Bryant, D.F., Cavanaugh, T. and Gange, T.A. (2003) 'The church: does it provide support for abused women? Differences in the perceptions of battered women and parishioners', *Journal of Religion and Abuse*, 5(1): 5–21.

Messina-Dysert, G. (2015) *Rape Culture and Spiritual Violence: religion, testimony and visions of healing*, London: Routledge.

Mitchell, J. (2012) *Promoting Peace, Inciting Violence: the role of religion and media*, London: Routledge.

Orr Macdonald, L. (2000) *Out of the Shadows: Christianity and violence against women in Scotland*, Edinburgh: Centre for Theology and Public Issues, University of Edinburgh.

Petersen, E. (2013) *I Am Woman, Episode 21, Season 2: Elizabeth Petersen*. Online. Available at www.iamwomanseries.com/our-stories/season-2-all-episodes/episode-21-elizabeth-petersen/ (accessed 11 January 2016).

Pew Research Center (2012) *The Global Religious Landscape: a report on the size and distribution of the world's major religious groups as of 2010*, Washington DC: Pew Research Center. Online. Available at www.pewforum.org/files/2014/01/global-religion-full.pdf (accessed 18 April 2016).

Rahim, H. (2000) 'Virtue, gender and the family: reflections on religious texts in Islam and Hinduism', *Journal of Social Distress and the Homeless*, 9(3): 187–99.

Shannon-Lewy, C. and Dull, V. (2005) 'The response of Christian clergy to domestic violence: help or hindrance?', *Aggression and Violent Behavior*, 10(6): 647–59.

SAFFI (South African Faith and Family Institute) (2014a) *Annual Report 2013–2014*. Online. Available at www.saffi.org.za/images/launch/downloads/4223%20saffi%20annual%20report%20Web.pdf (accessed 20 March 2015).

SAFFI (South African Faith and Family Institute) (2014b) *Take a Stand: faith leaders to address root causes of GBV*. Online. Available at www.saferspaces.org.za/blog/entry/take-a-stand-faith-leaders-pledge-to-address-root-causes-of-gbv (accessed 20 March 2015).

Strickland, G.A., Welshimer, K.I. and Sarvela, P.D. (1998) 'Clergy perspectives and practices regarding intimate violence: a rural view', *Journal of Rural Health*, 14(4): 305–11.

Timmerman, J.H. (1993) 'Religion and violence: the persistence of ambivalence', in E. Buchwald, P.R. Fletcher and M. Roth (eds) *Transforming a Rape Culture*, Minneapolis: Milkweed Editions.

Wendt, S. (2008) 'Christianity and domestic violence: feminist poststructuralist perspectives', *Affilia*, 23(2): 144–55.

West, T.C. (1999) *Wounds of the Spirit: black women, violence, and resistance ethics*, New York: New York University Press.

WCC (World Council of Churches) (2011) *Overcoming Violence: the ecumenical decade 2001–2010*, Geneva, World Council of Churches. Online. Available at www.overcoming-violence.org/fileadmin/dov/files/OvercomingViolence.pdf (accessed 22 August 2016).

WCC (World Council of Churches) (2016) *What is the World Council of Churches?* Online. Available at www.oikoumene.org/en/about-us (accessed 19 August 2016).

10

THE POTENTIAL CONTRIBUTION OF HEALTH AND SOCIAL CARE PROFESSIONAL PRACTICE TO PRIMARY PREVENTION

Ann Taket and Beth R. Crisp

Introduction

This chapter explores the potential contribution of the professional practice of health and social care staff to primary prevention of gender-based violence. We examine how the re-shaping of health professional practice in relation to areas of practice as diverse as mental health, disability, management of chronic conditions and HIV/AIDS care shares common features with what is identified as helpful practice in relation to responding to domestic violence. These features include ensuring that the consultation provides a safe space, is empowering to the patient, that the patient is regarded as a full partner in the decision-making process and respecting their autonomy. Such practice can be described as rights-based practice as well as person-centred. Moves towards person-centred practice with decision-making shared between patient and professional not only support the individual's autonomy in health and social care matters, but also offers a powerful experience of respectful relationships and joint decision-making that can contribute to each of the three areas identified as important for preventing gender-based violence, namely:

- promoting equal and respectful relationships between men and women;
- promoting non-violent social norms and reducing the effects of prior exposure to violence; and
- improving access to resources and systems of support.

This chapter begins by briefly overviewing the various user and social movements that have contributed to calls for person-centred practice within all health and social care settings. The second section then considers the human rights grounding for such practice, before the third section considers how person-centred care has been taken up in policy, practice and professional guidance. The chapter then moves on to consider the elements of person-centred care, and professional guidance on domestic violence, before comparing the two and examining how they can both contribute to primary prevention.

'Nothing about us without us'

Originating in Latin in fifteenth-century Central European political traditions (Davies 1984), the phrase 'Nothing about us without us' was taken up in English by disability rights activists in the 1990s according to Charlton (1998). Since then it has become associated with a wide range of different groups and social movements in relation to demands for participation in policy and practice settings. For example, it was used as the title of a 2008 manifesto produced by people who use drugs who participated in the consultations of a project on greater involvement of such individuals undertaken by the Canadian HIV/AIDS Legal Network, the Open Society Institute Public Health Program and the International HIV/AIDS Alliance (Nothing about Us without Us 2008), as well as of the report produced by the same three institutions which examines why it is important to increase meaningful involvement of people who use (or have used) illegal drugs in the response to HIV and hepatitis C, and how this can be done (Jürgens 2008). More recently it was the title of an editorial in the *American Medical Association's Journal of Ethics* in January 2016 about patient- and family-centred care (Paul 2016).

The right to participation

Human rights to participation are set out in many of the international treaties ratified by most countries. Article 25 in the International Covenant on Civil and Political Rights (ICCPR) recognises the right 'to take part in the conduct of public affairs', while Article 15 of the International Covenant on Economic, Social and Cultural Rights (ICESCR) recognises the right of everyone 'to take part in cultural life'. Participation is also closely involved in the 'right to health'.

The preamble to the World Health Organization (WHO) constitution talks about the 'right to health': 'the enjoyment of the highest attainable standard of health is one of the fundamental rights of every human being', while Article 25 of the Universal Declaration of Human Rights begins:

> Everyone has the right to a standard of living adequate for the health and well-being of himself and of his family, including foods, clothing, housing and medical care and necessary social services, and the right to security in the event of unemployment, sickness, disability, widowhood, old age or other lack of livelihood in circumstances beyond his control.

Article 12 in the ICESCR also covers the 'right to health', understood as the right of everyone to the enjoyment of the highest attainable standard of physical and mental health (the achievement of social health or wellbeing are assigned under other articles in the treaty). In the United Nations' *General Comment* that expands on the right to health (CESCR 2000), it is clearly set out that the right includes the right to participation in all health-related decision-making at all levels. Both the ICCPR and ICESCR highlight that such rights are to be enjoyed without discrimination (ICCPR, Article 2; ICESCR, Article 2), including that each member state agrees to undertake:

> to respect and to ensure to all individuals within its territory and subject to its jurisdiction the rights recognized in the present Covenant, without distinction of any kind, such as race, colour, sex, language, religion, political or other opinion, national or social origin, property, birth or other status.

Later treaties and accompanying guidance clarify that discrimination based on 'other status' includes that due to gender identity, sexuality, disability and aspects of health status such as being HIV positive or drug dependent.

Person-centred care in policy, practice and professional guidance

At the global level, the WHO promotes people-centredness as one of six attributes of health care quality, arguing that health care has become overly disease-focused and technology-driven and that medical education gives insufficient consideration to the psychosocial, emotional and cultural context of patients (WHO 2007): 'People-centred health care is rooted in universally held values and principles which are enshrined in international law, such as human rights and dignity, non-discrimination, participation and empowerment, access and equity, and a partnership of equals' (WHO 2007: 7). In May 2016 at the sixty-ninth World Health Assembly (WHA), member states adopted, with overwhelming support, resolution WHA 69.24 'Strengthening integrated people-centred health services' which supports the 'Framework on integrated people-centred health services' (WHO 2016). Within WHO (2016), the vision set out is one of the co-production of health, defined as:

> care that is delivered in an equal and reciprocal relationship between professionals, people using care services, their families and the communities to which they belong. It implies a long-term relationship between people, providers and health systems where information, decision-making and service delivery become shared.
>
> *(WHO 2016: 4)*

At the country level, policy and strategy statements and practice guidance also echo this support for person-centred care and shared decision-making, for example in Australia (Australian Commission on Safety and Quality in Health Care 2010), the UK (Department of Health 2007, 2010, 2013; NHS Education for Scotland 2011; NHS England 2013) and the US (US Government 2010). At state level in

Australia this is also the case (NSW Department of Health 2009; SA Health 2015; Victorian Department of Health 2012). At country level and below, a shift in terminology can be noticed in some cases, replacing 'person-centred' by 'patient-centred' or 'consumer-centred', both of which act to distance the concept from a basis in human rights.

Patient-centred care has also featured in many different sets of professional guidance for health and social care professionals. In the US, the Institute of Medicine (IOM) put forth patient-centred care as one of its six objectives for improving health care in the twenty-first century (IOM 2001). In the UK the General Dental Council's guidance for dental professionals recommends that patient-centred care principles should influence all areas of practice (GDC 2005). The General Medical Council's guidance on good medical practice (GMC 2013) does not explicitly mention patient-centred care; however, the duties of doctors that are included in the guidance include all the elements commonly identified with person-centred care.

The elements of person-centred care

There have been many different characterisations of the essential elements or components of person-centred care, those originating in the health sector usually substituting the term 'patient' for 'person'. Drawing on the Australian Commission on Safety and Quality in Health Care (2010), the Royal College of General Practitioners (2014), Hansson et al. (2015) and Mazurenko et al. (2015), Gluyas (2015: 50–1) emphasises the importance of recognising the uniqueness of each individual patient, and in responding to this, key elements of person-centred care are:

- providing emotional support and physical comfort;
- fostering a therapeutic relationship between the patient and health care professional team;
- sharing information, power and responsibility by engaging patients and their family and carers in the care process; and
- designing care processes to suit patient needs and ensure continuity of care.

(Gluyas 2015: 50–1)

A slightly different view is offered by the four principles of person-centred care put forward by the Health Foundation (2014: 6):

1. affording people dignity, compassion and respect;
2. offering coordinated care, support or treatment;
3. offering personalised care, support or treatment; and
4. supporting people to recognise and develop their own strengths and abilities to enable them to live an independent and fulfilling life.

Of particular interest is the fourth principle above, which others have characterised as an empowering approach (Foot et al. 2014; Pulvirenti et al. 2014), one element of which involves shared decision-making. To achieve this, particularly important characteristics required of the professional in person-centred care include: empathy, compassion, respect and a non-judgemental approach (WHO 2007; Health Foundation 2014; Scambler et al. 2015).

Guidance on domestic violence

Since the 1990s there has been an increasing number of publications containing professional guidance in relation to domestic violence, some profession-specific and others more general. This section explores some of the recent guidance from various different bodies and professional associations in health and social care. Some of these explicitly mention primary prevention. Most, however, are formulated in terms of responding to domestic violence rather than primary prevention. This section examines the potential for practice following this guidance to also serve a preventive function and compares the principles and professional characteristics involved with those set out above for person-centred care. Table 10.1 summarises some key features of the guidance documents considered, in terms of whether they explicitly mention primary prevention and whether they discuss a human rights grounding for the guidance.

As Table 10.1 shows, only three of the nine sets of guidance considered explicitly mention primary prevention, of which two (FVPF (Family Violence Prevention Fund) 2004; Fanslow et al. 2016) only mention the possibility. In the US national consensus guidelines on identifying and responding to domestic violence victimisation in health care settings, the section on definitions and rationale includes: 'Most Americans are seen at some point by a health care provider, and the health care setting offers a critical opportunity for early identification and even the primary prevention of abuse' (FVPF 2004: 2). New Zealand's 'Family Violence Assessment and Intervention Guideline' (Fanslow et al. 2016) talks about the potential primary prevention role of health care encounters through the reinforcement of healthy/respectful relationships as follows:

> As with other health care issues, health care providers have a continuum of options for their responses to relationship issues. For example:
>
> 1. If health care providers observe safe, stable and nurturing relationships between adults and children, and healthy/respectful relationships between adults, they can reinforce these through positive responses.
>
> *(Fanslow et al. 2016: 14)*

Turning to the third set of guidance that specifically mentions primary prevention (RACGP 2014), this discusses explicit examples of workplace-based strategies: respectful relationships and/or bystander training for staff; appointing practice/organisation champions who will institute prevention activities across the

TABLE 10.1 Selected recent guidance related to domestic violence

Country	Scope	Discussion of primary prevention	Explicit mention of rights	Reference
Global	Clinical and policy guidelines for health professionals	Not mentioned	Contains a section on the human rights underpinning of the guidelines	WHO 2013
Australia	General practice, primary care organisations	Yes, discusses concrete examples in the practice setting	Some consideration, but mostly in terms of groups like children, people with disabilities, refugees, etc.	RACGP 2014
Canada	Physician	Not mentioned	Not discussed explicitly	DOVE 2015
New Zealand	Health care settings	Yes, potential mentioned	Explicitly discussed	Fanslow et al. 2016
UK	General practice	Not mentioned	Not discussed explicitly	CAADA and IRIS 2012
UK	Multiagency work across health and social care	Not in health or social care settings	Not discussed explicitly	NICE 2014
UK	Medical professionals	Not in health settings	Some mention of rights	BMA Board of Science 2014
UK	Health and social care practitioners – quality standard	Not discussed	Not discussed	NICE 2016
US	Health care settings	Yes, potential mentioned	Not discussed explicitly	FVPF 2004

workplace; acknowledging significant days relating to the elimination of violence against women; and improving workplace climate and peer support for work in this area.

The global clinical and policy guidelines (WHO 2013) contain a section that explores the human rights underpinning of guidelines, while the New Zealand guidance (Fanslow et al. 2016) explicitly discusses rights issues throughout. Two other sets of guidance (BMA Board of Science 2014; RACGP 2014) contain some discussion of rights, but this is not a comprehensive treatment. The other sets of guidance do not discuss rights explicitly; however, the guidance contained is broadly consistent with a human rights framework.

In terms of supporting primary prevention, two further aspects are considered: the environment of the setting to which the guidance applies and the characterisation of the relationship between professional and client or patient. In both these cases what is set out in the guidance is highly consistent with providing support for what are considered three important strategies for preventing gender-based violence (VicHealth 2007, 2009), namely: promoting equal and respectful relationships between men and women; promoting non-violent social norms and reducing the effects of prior exposure to violence; and improving access to resources and systems of support.

First of all, considering the environment in the health or social care setting, this is explicitly considered in some professional guidance, for example in FVPF (2004), BMA Board of Science (2014), NICE (2014) and RACGP (2014). So, for example, as part of a recommendation for creating an environment for disclosing domestic violence and abuse, NICE (2014) states:

> Health and social care service managers and managers of specialist domestic violence and abuse services and related services should:
>
> - Clearly display information in waiting areas and other suitable places about the support on offer for those affected by domestic violence and abuse. This includes contact details of relevant local and national helplines. It could also include information for groups who may find it more difficult to disclose that they are experiencing violence and abuse . . . .
> - Ensure the information on where to get support is available in a range of formats and locally used languages. The former could include braille and audio versions and the use of large font sizes. There may also be more discreet ways of conveying information, for example, by providing pens or key rings with a helpline number.
>
> *(NICE 2014: 12)*

FVPF (2004) suggests, in addition, 'Have brochures placed in exam rooms and private places such as bathrooms' (FVPF 2004: 57), and emphasises the importance, wherever information is provided, of including information about victims/survivors, perpetrators and the impact of domestic violence on children. As the various different guidance explains, displaying such information contributes to reinforcing that domestic violence is wrong and unacceptable, and works to change public perceptions of domestic violence, reinforce non-violent social norms and promote equal and respectful relationships, thus contributing to primary prevention.

Turning now to the interaction between professionals and patients or clients, all of the guidance discusses the important characteristics of these relationships in similar terms, emphasising the importance of empathy, compassion, sensitivity, respect and being non-judgemental. RACGP (2014) expresses it as follows:

Respect is an overarching principle when dealing with issues of abuse and violence. This involves respecting patient's wishes, respecting our own limits and abilities to undertake abuse and violence work and, finally, modelling respectful relationships with our colleagues and in the community.

(RACGP 2014: 122)

This implicitly recognises the importance of professionals' contribution to primary prevention in terms of modelling respectful relationships.

The characteristics of relationships between professional and clients/patients described in domestic violence guidance are broadly the same as those described earlier in this chapter for person-centred care; they are also mirrored in what is found from qualitative studies of women regarding the characteristics they would like to see in their relationships with health professionals when discussing domestic violence (Feder et al. 2006). It is important to note one difference between person-centred care and domestic violence related consultations, namely that person-centred care is usually couched in terms of joint decision-making, whereas guidance for consultations around domestic violence strongly emphasise respecting the woman's autonomy to make her own decisions.

Supporting primary prevention

Siloed funding agreements can readily lead to organisations that are not explicitly funded to undertake primary prevention of family violence failing to recognise the contributions they can make in this area. For example, the provision of services to address mental health or substance misuse (Dennis 2014; Hartney and Barnard 2015) or poverty (Hart 2008) can be effective forms of primary prevention. Similarly, detailed individual position descriptions, which make no mention of preventive work, can readily lead staff members to consider prevention as something which is the responsibility of others. Organisations that are most effectively engaged in prevention work are those which are

focusing on activities that achieve a real difference, using evidence of results to improve performance, making good use of resources, and being ambitious to solve problems. This requires high-quality leadership and staff, and good financial management.

(van Poortvliet 2012: 18)

There may be times when organisations need to reconsider operating practices, where these are obstructing them from achieving their key objectives. For example, if an organisation is obsessed with cleanliness and order, parents with young children may feel unwelcome and not establish and maintain supportive relationships which have preventive potential (Erickson et al. 2014). New mothers experiencing domestic violence were up to six times more likely to have discontinued participation in a home visiting service by the time their child was six months of age than new mothers who were not experiencing violence (Flemington and Fraser 2016). However, while it may be tempting to assume that family violence leads to mothers disengaging with programmes, another possibility is that 'building mothers' resilience and coping strategies is an important preventive task' (Dennis 2014: 30).

In families where there is a complex array of stresses and problems, inadequate support overall, short-term provision and fragmented services that are contradictory in their approach may exacerbate the potential for family violence. However, complex interventions, while initially expensive, can actually be cost effective in the longer term (van Poortvleit 2012). In guidance prepared for philanthropic organisations in the UK, it has been proposed that:

> Funders should therefore prioritise service delivery and expansion of effective programmes. They should focus on preventing problems before they emerge and on ensuring that effective models retain quality and work with the highest need families. They should also try to meet gaps – whether geographical gaps in services funded by government, or gaps in the types of service provided, such as mental health support.
>
> *(van Poortvliet 2012: 14)*

Health and social care staff need to be able to recognise the potential for family violence caused by a wide range of stresses on individuals and families, and not just where violence has previously occurred or been threatened in respect of persons, property or pets. In particular, they must also ensure they do not inadvertently put women at risk by enabling their whereabouts to be discovered by persons who may cause them harm. This not only includes keeping addresses and other contact details secure, but considering whether passing a present on to a child might lead to discovery if a tracking device was hidden in the gift (Queensland Law Society 2016).

Working effectively to prevent family violence can require professionals to reconsider what may have been accepted practice within their professions. Professional supervision and ongoing professional development are recommended, if not mandatory, for many health and social care professionals, and can be critical in ensuring experienced practitioners are aware of emerging critiques of what was once status quo thinking (Grealy et al. 2008). For example, when the second author studied to become a social worker in the 1980s, systems theory was far more fashionable than it is now within Australian schools of social work. However, if systems theory is to be appropriately applied in prevention of family violence, alternative understandings of how this can be used may be required:

> A major criticism of systemic approaches to counselling practice from a family violence perspective is that they potentially shift responsibility for the violence away from the perpetrator. Violence can be positioned as occurring because of the nature and structure of the family or the dynamics within that system, placing 'blame' for violence on all members of that unit rather than the perpetrator. While a systemic approach may be useful in terms of

understanding violence as something that occurs within the context of a family unit, the unequal power relationships within a family violence situation can't be ignored. Systems theory must be applied with reference to the basic safety of women and children who are experiencing violence, and in a way that ensures the counselling process does not divert responsibility for the violence from the perpetrator.

(Grealy et al. 2008: 25)

For those of us involved in the formation of health and social care clinicians, our contributions to eliminating gender-based violence do not just consist of the theories and methods we teach. Rather, the role of educators is to ensure that health and social care graduates understand that taking preventive measures is not considered less important compared with the pressures of responding to incidents of gender-based violence (Crisp and Beddoe 2013). Thus,

education optimally needs more focus on the interacting factors which contribute to an individual's health, well-being and resources, where there may be no obvious risk of immediate harm but where well-being and quality of life is threatened.

(Coren et al. 2011: 595)

Increasing opportunities for primary prevention

This chapter has explored the potential contribution of the professional practice of health and social care staff to primary prevention of gender-based violence. It has demonstrated how the moves to person-centred care and improved response to domestic violence as encapsulated in professional guidance are mutually reinforcing and serve to put professionals in a position to model respectful relationships and reinforce non-violent social norms, a very important part of primary prevention.

It has also illustrated how the broader environment in which health and social care settings operate has an important role to play in primary prevention. This includes the priority setting of funding organisations, the role of higher education in effectively equipping graduates to recognise prevention as integral to their work, and the management of health and social care services. Looking ahead as health and social care services around the globe push forward in terms of implementing person-centred care and developing the service response to domestic violence and abuse, such moves will also increase the contribution to primary prevention that can be made in health and social care settings.

References

Australian Commission on Safety and Quality in Health Care (2010) *Patient-Centred Care: improving quality and safety through partnerships with patients and consumers,* Sydney: Australian Commission on Safety and Quality in Health Care.

BMA Board of Science (2014) *Domestic Abuse*, London: British Medical Association.

CAADA and IRIS (2012) *Responding to Domestic Abuse: guidance for general practices*, London: RCGP and NSPCC.

CESCR (2000) *General Comment No. 14: the right to the highest attainable standard of health*, Geneva: United Nations.

Charlton, J.I. (1998) *Nothing about Us without Us*, San Francisco: University of California Press.

Coren, E., Iredale, W., Rutter, D. and Bywaters, P. (2011) 'The contribution of social work and social interventions across the life course to the reduction of health inequalities: a new agenda for social work education?', *Social Work Education*, 30: 594–609.

Crisp, B.R. and Beddoe, L. (2013) 'Conclusion: developing an agenda to promote health and well-being in social work education', in B.R. Crisp and L. Beddoe (eds) *Promoting Health and Well-being in Social Work Education*, London: Routledge.

Davies, N. (1984). *Heart of Europe: the past in Poland's present*, Oxford: Oxford University Press.

Dennis, T. (2014) 'Time to tackle domestic violence: identifying and supporting families', *Community Practitioner*, 87(9): 29–32.

Department of Health (2007) *Putting People First: a shared vision and commitment to the transformation of adult social care*, London: The Stationery Office.

Department of Health (2010) *Equity and Excellence: liberating the NHS. Cm 7881*, London: The Stationery Office.

Department of Health (2013) *Treating Patients and Service Users with Respect, Dignity and Compassion*. Online. Available at http://tinyurl.com/q3ew7a6 (accessed 7 May 2014).

DOVE (2015) *Towards Optimised Practice: clinical practice guideline, domestic violence*, Canadian Medical Association. Online. Available at www.cma.ca/En/Pages/cpg-by-condition.aspx?conditionCode=1641 (accessed 4 February 2017).

Erickson, C.L., Gault, D. and Simmons, D. (2014) '"The Wakanheza Project": a public health approach to primary prevention of family violence', *Journal of Community Practice*, 22: 67–81.

FVPF (Family Violence Prevention Fund) (2004) *National Consensus Guidelines on Identifying and Responding to Domestic Violence Victimization in Health Care Settings*, San Francisco: Family Violence Prevention Fund.

Fanslow, J.L., Kelly. P. and Ministry of Health (2016) *Family Violence Assessment and Intervention Guideline: child abuse and intimate partner violence*, 2nd edn, Wellington: Ministry of Health.

Feder, G.S., Hutson, M., Ramsay, J. and Taket, A.R. (2006) 'Women exposed to intimate partner violence, expectations and experiences when they encounter healthcare professionals: a meta-analysis of qualitative studies', *Archives of Internal Medicine*, 166: 12–37.

Flemington, T. and Fraser, J.A. (2016) 'Maternal involvement in a nurse home visiting programme to prevent child maltreatment', *Journal of Children's Services*, 11: 124–40.

Foot, C., Gilburt, H., Dunn, P., Jabbal, J., Seale, B., Goodrich. J., Buck, D. and Taylor, J. (2014) *People in Control of their own Health and Care: the state of involvement*, London: The King's Fund in association with National Voices.

GDC (2005) *General Dental Council Standard Guidance*, London: GDC.

GMC (General Medical Council) (2013) *Good Medical Practice: working with doctors, working for patients*, London: GMC.

Gluyas, H. (2015) 'Patient-centred care: improving healthcare outcomes', *Nursing Standard*, 30(4): 50–9.

Grealy, C., Humphreys, C., Milward, K. and Power, J. (2008) *Practice Guidelines: women's and children's family violence counselling and support program*, Melbourne: Department of Human Services, Victoria.

Hansson, E., Ekman, I., Swedberg, K., Wolf, A., Dudas, K. Ehlers, L. and Olsson L.-E. (2015) 'Person-centred care for patients with chronic heart failure – a cost–utility analysis', *European Journal of Cardiovascular Nursing*, 15: 276–84.

Hart, D. (2008) 'Trapped within poverty and violence', in B. Fawcett and F. Waugh (eds) *Addressing Violence, Abuse and Oppression: debates and challenges*, London: Routledge.

Hartney, E. and Barnard, D.K. (2015) 'A framework for the prevention and mitigation of injury from family violence in children of parents with mental illness and substance use problems', *Aggression and Violent Behavior*, 25: 354–62.

Health Foundation (2014) *Person-Centred Care Made Simple*, London: Health Foundation.

IOM (Institute of Medicine) (2001) *Crossing the Quality Chasm: a new health system for the 21st century*, Washington, DC: National Academy Press.

Jürgens, R, (2008) *'Nothing about Us without Us': greater, meaningful involvement of people who use illegal drugs: a public health, ethical, and human rights imperative*, International edition, Toronto: Canadian HIV/AIDS Legal Network, International HIV/AIDS Alliance, Open Society Institute.

Mazurenko, O., Bock, S., Prato, C. and Bondarenko, M. (2015) 'Considering shared power and responsibility: diabetic patients' experience with the PCMH care model', *Journal of Patient Experience*, 2: 61–7.

NHS Education for Scotland (2011) *Quality Education for a Healthier Scotland – Strategic Framework: 2011–2014*, Edinburgh: NHS Education for Scotland.

NHS England (2013) *Putting Patients First: The NHS England business plan for 2013/14– 2015/16*, London: The Stationery Office.

NICE (National Institute for Health and Care Excellence) (2014) *Domestic Violence and Abuse: how health services, social care and the organisations they work with can respond effectively. NICE Public Health Guidance 50*, London: NICE.

NICE (2016) *Domestic Violence and Abuse: quality standard*. Online. Available at www.nice.org. uk/guidance/qs116 (accessed 1 March 2017).

Nothing about Us without Us (2008) *Nothing about Us without Us, a Manifesto by People Who Use Illegal Drugs*, Canadian HIV/AIDS Legal Network, the International HIV/AIDS Alliance, and the Open Society Institute. Online. Available at www.opensocietyfounda-tions.org/reports/nothing-about-us-without-us (accessed 24 February 2017).

NSW Department of Health (2009) *Working with Essentials of Care: a resource guide for facilita-tors*, Sydney: NSW Department of Health.

Paul, T. (2016) '"Nothing about us without us": toward patient- and family-centered care', *AMA Journal of Ethics*, 18: 3–5.

Pulvirenti, M., McMillan, J. and Lawn, S. (2014) 'Empowerment, patient centred care and self-management', *Health Expectations*: 17: 303–10.

Queensland Law Society (2016) *Domestic and Family Violence: best practice guidelines*, Brisbane: Queensland Law Society. Online. Available at www.qls.com.au/for_the_profession/advo-cacy/domestic_and_family_violence_best_practice_guidelines (accessed 9 March 2017).

RACGP (2014) *Abuse and Violence: working with our patients in general practice*, 4th edn, Melbourne: Royal Australian College of General Practitioners.

Royal College of General Practitioners (2014) *An Inquiry into Patient Centred Care in the 21st Century: implications for general practice and primary care*, London: Royal College of General Practitioners.

SA Health (2015) *Delivering Transforming Health*, Adelaide, South Australia: Department for Health and Ageing, Government of South Australia.

Scambler, S., Gupta, A. and Asimakopoulou, K. (2015) 'Patient-centred care – what is it and how is it practised in the dental surgery?', *Health Expectations*, 18: 2549–58.

US Government (2010) *Patient Protection and Affordable Care Act (PPACA) HR3590*, Washington, DC: US Government Publishing Office.

van Poortvliet, M. (2012) *Out of Trouble: families with complex problems. A guide for funders*, London: New Philanthropy Capital. Online. Available at www.thinknpc.org/publications/out-of-trouble-2/ (accessed 9 March 2017).

VicHealth (2007) *Preventing Violence Before it Occurs: a framework and background paper to guide the primary prevention of violence against women in Victoria*, Carlton: Victorian Health Promotion Foundation.

VicHealth (2009) *Preventing Violence Before it Occurs: a framework for action*, Carlton: Victorian Health Promotion Foundation.

Victorian Department of Health (2012) *Best Care for Older People Everywhere: the toolkit*, Melbourne: Government of Victoria.

WHO (2007) *People-Centred Health Care: a policy framework*, Geneva: WHO, Western Pacific Region.

WHO (2013) *Responding to Intimate Partner Violence and Sexual Violence against Women: WHO clinical and policy guidelines*, Geneva: WHO.

WHO (2016) *Framework on Integrated People-Centred Health Services. Sixty-ninth World Health Assembly, Provisional agenda item 16.1 A69/39*. Geneva: WHO.

11

ASSET-BASED APPROACHES FOR PREVENTING GENDER-BASED VIOLENCE IN THE WORKPLACE

Beth R. Crisp and Ann Taket

Introduction

Gender-based violence (GBV) impacts not only on those who are directly targeted for abuse, but on those people and environments with which they are in regular contact (Riger et al. 2002). This includes workplaces. Indeed, the impact of GBV in the workplace has long been recognised and it is now two decades since Joy Mighty, discussing the Canadian context, wrote:

> In the same way that employers have a social responsibility to conduct business in ways that protect the environment, they also have a social responsibility to create a workplace environment that gives the clear message that any form of violence against female (or male) employees is not to be tolerated.
>
> *(Mighty 1997: 256)*

Historically, one of the ways employers responded to intimate partner violence (IPV) was to terminate the employment of women experiencing violence (Riger et al. 2000; Shepard and Pence 1988; Swanberg et al. 2006). There is now increasing recognition of the need to support women experiencing IPV (Swanberg et al. 2012). However, this often involves organisations responding to employees who have disclosed their status as victims of IPV (Swanberg and Logan 2005; Swanberg et al. 2006; Versola-Russo and Russo 2009) rather than proactive efforts to reduce the likelihood of such violence occurring in the first place. Furthermore, this makes it difficult for employers to provide support as many women will not disclose to their employers (Swanberg et al. 2005). Hence, this chapter explores the benefits for employers in promoting strategies to 'promote respectful and equitable relationships' (Chung et al. 2012: 35) both within and beyond the organisation as their part of broader societal efforts to eliminate GBV.

How does challenging GBV benefit employers?

There are good reasons for employers to recognise the impact (actual or potential) of GBV in the workplace. In terms of making a case as to why an organisation should invest in violence-prevention work, this can include statements as to why this is relevant to core business, cost–benefit analysis, a way of demonstrating organisational core values and enhancing reputation in the wider community (Upston and Durey 2012). Therefore, irrespective of whether employers consider that they have a moral duty to tackle GBV, from an asset-management perspective, this may make good sense. In addition to the costs incurred to individual survivors and their families, the economic consequences for workplaces are increasingly realised as there are impacts on capacity to work for almost all victims of GBV (Swanberg and Logan 2005).

As far back as 1995, it was estimated that 13.5 million work days were lost in the US alone due to intimate partner violence (Max et al. 2004). The cost of domestic violence in Australia in 2014–15 was estimated to be A\$21.7 billion, of which 6 per cent or A\$1.3 billion were costs experienced by employers (PricewaterhouseCoopers 2015). These costs include lowered productivity, increased sick leave, increased workplace injuries, and higher costs associated with staff turnover and recruitment (Moe and Bell 2004; Swanberg et al. 2005; Upston and Durey 2012).

Absence from work is costly for employers as victims of GBV often need to take time off or may not be able to retain their employment (Browne et al. 1999). In the short term, they may be injured or too ill to attend work (Swanberg et al. 2006) and there can be ongoing loss of productivity if the health impacts remain long term (Reeves and O'Leary-Kelly 2007). Victims may also be prevented from going to work, through tactics such as sabotaging a car or stealing car keys or money for transport to get to work (Swanberg et al. 2006). Alternatively, they may arrive late or need to leave early due to reasons associated with IPV (Reeves and O'Leary-Kelly 2007; Swanberg et al. 2005). Family members or friends also may need to take time off to support victims of GBV (Upston and Durey 2012).

In addition to absence due to GBV, there are also the problems associated with workers who are present but underperforming or unable to perform some tasks because of distractions (Reeves and O'Leary-Kelly 2007; Versola-Russo and Russo 2009; Upston and Durey 2012). In particular, victims of IPV may have their capacity to work undermined if the abuse follows them to the workplace in the form of harassment or surveillance of employees by perpetrators, and seeking them out in the workplace (Wathen et al. 2016). This can occur through the perpetrator turning up to the workplace in person or by other means such as telephone (Lloyd and Taluc 1999). For victims who have moved house to get away from perpetrators, workplaces may be one of the places where they can be readily located by a former partner (Swanberg et al. 2005). Consequently, violence from partners is a leading cause of death for women in the workplace and may also impact on the safety of others there (Swanberg et al. 2005; Wathen et al. 2016).

Employees have a right to a safe workplace, and employers have a duty of care to provide this (Swanberg et al. 2012):

> Other people on the workplace premises, including supervisors, other work-ers, and customers, are at risk for injury or some other form of trauma. As such, workplaces could benefit from implementing various procedures to deal with partner violence as a separate form of workplace violence.
>
> *(Swanberg et al. 2006: 573)*

Not only does IPV cause problems for the employers of victims, it can also be problematic for the workplaces of perpetrators. As with victims, perpetrators may demonstrate impaired job performance and less productivity (Mankowski et al. 2013). Perpetrators miss more work than their colleagues (Rothman and Corso 2008) and when they are at work may be using workplace resources to perpetrate IPV. This includes use of telephone, email and company vehicles for surveillance (Galvez et al. 2011; Rothman and Perry 2004). Perpetrators also make more mis-takes at work than their colleagues (Rothman and Corso 2008), which may be extremely costly both in direct financial terms and in loss of reputation (Murray and Powell 2007; Rothman and Perry 2004), as well as compromise workplace safety (Mankowski et al. 2013).

Workplace initiatives to confront GBV

Workplace programmes which work with perpetrators to tackle IPV are a relatively recent innovation and typically provide support to perpetrators who self-identify this as a problem (Walters et al. 2012). Such is their newness that a recent systematic review of economic costs associated with prevention programmes does not iden-tify any workplace initiatives (PricewaterhouseCoopers 2015). However, workplace initiatives which explicitly seek to confront IPV will have at best limited potential in facilitating change. Many perpetrators do not acknowledge their violent acts and would not come to the notice of workplace programmes even if they did exist (Walters et al. 2012). Nevertheless, whether or not they have disclosed to their employers, perpetrators of IPV may often display aggressive or other inappropriate behaviours in the workplace (Rothman and Perry 2004).

Although programmes which explicitly target IPV have been found to result in changes in attitude and/or behaviours towards women by some men, these programmes typically require male participants to identify themselves as being the problem and hence needing to change. Furthermore, by focusing on chang-ing individual behaviours and encouraging rejection of attitudes and behaviours which perpetuate violence against women, deficit-based approaches run the risk of blaming and alienating those individuals whose behaviour is regarded as most problematic.

A potentially more effective way to engage with issues of GBV in the work-place is to engage with the wider workforce around issues of gender equity and hence 'overcome resistance and defensiveness' of perpetrators and 'decrease victim-blaming messages whether intentional or not' (Banyard et al. 2004: 66–7). Hence, workplace approaches are particularly likely to be well-received in organisations in which staff perceive their line managers and close colleagues as strongly disapproving of gender-based violence (Cunradi et al. 2008). For example, when 600 staff from Linfox, a transport and logistics business with predominantly male staff, participated in workplace training around gender equity and violence prevention, 95 per cent of participants were reportedly pleased the programme had been provided in their workplaces (Upston and Durey 2012)

Furthermore, IPV is not the only manifestation of gender-based violence in the workplace. In recent years it has become common practice within workplaces to establish policies and procedures to deal with issues such as sexual harassment, bullying and ensuring that one's gender is not a barrier to realising ambitions associated with employment (Swanberg et al. 2012). A common factor across these issues is inequalities in the distribution of power and resources (Our Watch et al. 2015; VicHealth 2007; Wall 2014).

Gender stereotyping often occurs within organisations but assumptions about gender tend not to be articulated until challenged (Barnett 2004; Kugelberg 2006). Consequently, many organisations continue to operationalise gendered assumptions which confirm and perpetuate gendered norms in their work practices (Ely and Myerson 2010). In the extreme, this can result in a situation in which the

> definition of manhood is a man *in* power, a man *with* power, and a man *of* power. We equate manhood with being strong, successful, capable, reliable, in control. The very definitions of manhood we have developed in our culture maintain the power that some men have over other men and that men have over women.
>
> *(Kimmel 1994: 125)*

It has been argued that until such assumptions that result in gender inequity are recognised and practices changed, tackling issues such as IPV cannot occur in more than a token manner (Swanberg 2004). Hence, primary prevention approaches to reducing violence against women are now tending to focus on improving gender equity more broadly by promoting and/or modelling attitudes and behaviours which promote gender equity (Fleming et al. 2015). Such efforts capitalise on the capacity of workplaces to model positive behaviours in regard to respectful relationships and promoting an ethos of gender equity, as well as challenging problematic beliefs associated with violence and abuse (Upston and Durey 2012).

Identifying and removing barriers to women's participation and leadership in the workplace is one of many strategies which contribute to gender equity. Furthermore, in order to sustain changes by individuals in their attitudes and behaviours, cultural change is also required. This may include the introduction of policies and procedures which promote gender equity and take a stance against practices that have allowed discrimination or harassment of women to become embedded within organisations (Dyson and Flood 2008: 17). As such, efforts to promote gender equity are not only inclusive but consistent with asset-based approaches which seek to maximise the effectiveness of the workforce (Chung et al. 2012; Dyson and Flood 2008; VicHealth 2013). Moreover, workplaces have been identified as strategic settings for the promotion of health and wellbeing more generally (WHO 2010). Hence, efforts to improve gender equity at an organisational level contribute to broader community efforts to promote a culture of respect in which gender-based violence is not tolerated (Chung et al. 2012; Holmes and Flood 2013).

Implementing workplace programmes

Preventing violence against women in any setting, including workplaces, requires a multi-strategy approach, ideally involving strategies that are contemporaneous (Fleming et al. 2015). For instance, there is little point in an organisation engaging in efforts at primary prevention and at the same time failing to respond to incidents of violence or harassment in the workplace, or not having the capacity to recognise how entrenched policies and procedures in the workplace may be contributing to gender inequity (Chung et al. 2012). Moreover, efforts to combat gender inequity are much more likely to be effective as part of overall cultural change which seeks to challenge other common forms of disadvantage and discrimination, such as class, disability, ethnicity, religion and sexual identity (Our Watch et al. 2015; Wall 2014).

The initiatives described below were part of a much larger programme of work, namely a strategy for preventing violence against women and children in the north-east region of the state of Victoria, Australia. The overall programme had the following objectives:

1. to establish partnerships across government and non-government agencies as well as accountable leadership structures for sustainable prevention;
2. to support organisations to provide structural and cultural environments that promote equal and respectful relations;
3. to build the capacity of leaders to take action against sexism and rigid gender roles, and promote organisational change and workforce development;
4. to promote and communicate key messages and tools that build respectful relationships skills and influence social norms, attitudes and behaviours;
5. to undertake research, evaluation and monitoring to ensure continuous improvement and contribute to the evidence base.

(Taket et al. 2016: 88)

Commencing in 2014, two organisations within the region trialled programmes of work with a specific focus on improving gender equity. While both organisations provide services to dispersed rural communities from multiple service points and are in areas in which both agriculture and tourism are key industries, Alpine Health provides a range of health promotion, primary care and inpatient services, whereas Murrindindi Shire Council is a local government authority. The geography of the region would render it very unlikely that an individual was simultaneously employed by and/or using the services of both organisations.

Violence prevention programmes in the workplace are most likely to succeed if seen to be supported by senior management endorsing the initiatives and making it known that they believe them to be beneficial for their organisations (Upston and Durey 2012). Furthermore, not only is management support vital, a nominated group to oversee and coordinate efforts is crucial (Noblet and LaMontagne 2009). Such commitments were made in both organisations.

As effective programmes take into account the specific characteristics of an organisation and have the flexibility to be implemented in a way that recognises these factors (Noblet and LaMontagne 2009; Upston and Durey 2012), work commenced in both organisations through a gender audit conducted using the *Interaction Gender Audit Tool* (Harvey and Morris 2010) as the basis for developing an evidence-based gender action plan. To encourage ownership of the action plan, opportunities to contribute included completing surveys, participating in focus groups and being involved in the working group which was guiding the process in each organisation.

A short survey of gender attitudes was administered in both organisations over a three-month period in late 2014/early 2015. The survey items were based on questions which form the Gender Equity Scale which was used in the National Community Attitudes towards Violence against Women Survey (NCAS) conducted in Australia in 2009 and 2013 (McGregor 2009; Webster et al. 2014) as well as questions from the British Cohort Study (1996).

Almost three-quarters (72 per cent) of Murrindindi staff responded to the baseline survey about gender equity (Modderman 2015b) compared with one-third of staff (33 per cent) at Alpine Health (Modderman 2015a), with this lower participation rate likely to be an effect of organisational changes occurring at the time. Anecdotal reports suggest the survey respondents were representative of the gender mix profile in each organisation's staff profile (Taket et al. 2016). Whereas initiatives labelled as 'prevention of men's violence against women' may alienate some staff (Kilgower 2014), both organisations presented the work under the banner of 'gender equity'.

Organisational initiatives to promote gender equity included use of enterprise agreements as a platform for making statements about gender equity and incorporating prevention of domestic violence into human resources policies, including those associated with workplace behaviour, harassment and bullying (Upston and Durey 2012). Staff in both organisations were also given the opportunity to contribute their ideas about the development of a gender equity plan and their views as to what it would mean to be working in a gender-sensitive organisation, through participating in focus groups. Whereas in Alpine Health the need most commonly discussed was the need for all staff to be respected irrespective of gender (Büsst 2015a), staff at Murrindindi were also concerned with ensuring equitable access and selection on merit to positions, as well as prevention of family violence through developing greater understandings of gender equity (Büsst 2015b). Staff in both organisations recognised that such changes do not emerge just because they are desired but may require additional information and provision of relevant training.

In Alpine Health, the 'Respect and Equity Plan' was developed between July and September 2015 and included: the development of a gender equity procedure and of a gender equity lens for review of policies and procedures; provision of training and leadership programmes; communication to staff through regular newsletters; and setting up an annual review and reporting on the plan. The plan recognised that training and other activities needed to be provided during paid time, with an expectation of staff attendance (Upston and Durey 2012). Hence, bystander training workshops for staff were run in October 2015, while preparatory work for implementation of other items in the plan was being undertaken from November 2015.

At Murrindindi Shire Council, the action plan developed in July and August 2015 and implemented from December that year included a focus on disseminating what the organisation was already doing to enhance gender equity, with a new 'Did you know …?' poster or information sheet to be produced each month. However, it was also recognised that organisational policies and practices may be hindering attempts at gender equity. Hence, two major reviews of practice and procedure in the organisation included scrutiny to ensure gender equity and specific actions as required to embed these. Such actions included reviewing recruitment, induction and mentoring of new staff, professional development and training provided to all staff, and ensuring forms and templates were not biased towards one gender.

In late 2015, the gender equity surveys were readministered. Table 11.1 shows views on items associated with gender equity for pre- and post-implementation data in both organisations. As high levels of gender equity are represented by agreeing to some questions and disagreeing with others, items are presented such that the highest possible score of 100 represents complete gender equity, and the lowest possible score of zero represents complete gender inequity.

In both organisations, higher scores of gender equity in the post-implementation data were recorded for the majority of the 11 items. However, while there were increases recorded on nine items at Murrindindi, positive changes towards gender equity were found for only six items for staff at Alpine Health. Nevertheless, statistical testing of the pre- and post-implementation item scores for each organisation revealed no significant changes had occurred over time.

As the first eight items in Table 11.1 reflect items in the NCAS, a gender equity score for each respondent was calculated using the process utilised by Webster et al. (2014) in their analysis of the 2013 NCAS data. This yields a score of between 5 and 100, in which scores are classified as 'high' (greater than 90), 'medium' (75 to 90) and 'low' (less than 75). (See Table 11.2.)

In both organisations there was a positive change over time but the differences were not statistically significant. The post-implementation data from Murrindindi revealed a similar level of attitudes to gender equity as had been found in the 2013 NCAS. While higher levels of attitudes to gender equity were found at Alpine Health in the second data collection, this emerges from higher baseline data. Such

TABLE 11.1 Changes in gender attitudes pre- and post-implementation of survey in Alpine Health and Murrindindi Shire Council

	Alpine Health		Murrindini	
	Pre	Post	Pre	Post
In general, men make better political leaders than women (disagree)	57.1	77.5	61.4	47.1
When jobs are scarce men should have more right to a job than women (disagree)	91.3	97.5	75.0	88.3
A university education is more important for a boy than a girl (disagree)	96.1	97.5	80.7	82.4
A woman has to have children to be fulfilled (disagree)	91.3	85.0	80.7	82.3
It's OK for a woman to have a child as a single parent and not want a stable relationship with a man (agree)	61.9	62.5	52.3	76.5
Discrimination against women is no longer a problem in the workplace in Australia (disagree)	85.8	90.0	72.7	82.3
Men should take control in relationships and be the head of the household (disagree)	85.7	85.0	68.2	58.9
Women prefer a man to be in charge of the relationship (disagree)	80.2	77.5	63.6	82.4
There should be more women in senior management positions in business and industry (agree)	62.7	70.0	52.3	64.7
When both partners work full-time, they should have equal share of domestic chores (agree)	92.1	72.5	77.3	94.1
If a child is ill and both parents are working, it should usually be the mother who takes time off work to look after the child (disagree)	66.6	57.5	59.1	70.6
N	126	40	88	17

Source: Compiled from pages 36, 37, 41 and 42 of Taket et al. (2016).

TABLE 11.2 Percentage of individuals by level of gender equity scores for Alpine Health, Murrindindi Shire Council and the NCAS 2013 sample

Gender Equity Score	Alpine Health		Murrindindi		NCAS 2013
	Pre	Post	Pre	Post	
High	50.8	57.5	30.7	35.5	34.3
Medium	38.1	37.5	38.6	41.2	42.6
Low	11.1	5.0	30.7	23.5	23.1
N	126	40	88	17	17,495

Source: Compiled from Table 14 (page 41) and Table 15 (page 46) of Taket et al. (2016).

differences in the baseline data support the initial contention that different strategies might be require for each organisation.

As the post-implementation data collection occurred at a point when implementation of the action plans had only just begun, the changes from the baseline may in fact assess the impact of the baseline survey in encouraging individual staff to review their views on matters associated with gender equity. The response rates for the post-implementation data was 19 per cent for Murrindindi Shire Council and 11 per cent at Alpine Health. In both organisations there was possibly a perception that it was too soon to be doing a follow-up survey, especially given the lack of time for the action plan implementation to have had much impact on staff.

To encourage participation in the surveys, information which might have enabled identification of an individual employee was not collected. Therefore, it was not possible to match individual responses collected at pre-implementation with those collected post-implementation. Consequently, it was also not possible to determine how many post-implementation respondents had previously completed the baseline survey. Nor has it been possible to explore the representativeness of any sample, apart from the gender profile, in respect to the overall workforce in each organisation.

Discussion

Achieving gender-based equity in the workplace remains a challenge, even when staff are committed to it. However, this does not mean that gender equity should cease to be an organisational aim, but rather that we should recognise that this is not something which can be rapidly achieved and ticked off as no longer an issue (Seymour 2009).

While the majority of the changes between the baseline and post-implementation surveys in both workplaces discussed here are in a positive direction, the magnitude of changes was not statistically significant in either organisation. Nevertheless, subsequent anecdotal reports support the trends to higher levels of gender equity found in the quantitative data and suggest that organisations can model alternative behaviours which promote gender equity (Ely and Myerson 2010).

Importantly, data collected from the baseline surveys was not for the evaluation of the initiatives, but along with focus groups and other sources, contributed to an evidence-based participative process to produce an action plan tailored to the specific needs of each organisation. While these action plans included primary prevention initiatives, secondary and tertiary components, such as establishing policies and procedures to respond to sexual harassment or violence, may also have a primary preventive effect on social norms and organisational culture (Chung et al. 2012). Building collective ownership of gender equity plans and initiatives to prevent gender-based violence also limits the potential for ongoing implementation to cease should a key staff member leave the organisation (Murray and Powell 2007).

The asset-based approaches to violence prevention as described in this chapter coincided with a growing recognition in the wider Australian community that gender-based violence was a serious problem which must be addressed. However, while it is not possible to determine the extent to which the broader context was an enabler of changes to organisational processes or culture, organisations embarking on this process where the broader context is not so supportive may find the process more challenging.

References

Banyard, V., Plante, E. and Moynihan, M. (2004) 'Bystander education: bringing a broader perspective to sexual violence prevention', *Journal of Community Psychology*, 32(1): 61–79.

Barnett, R.C. (2004) 'Preface: women and work: where are we, where did we come from, and where are we going?', *Journal of Social Issues*, 60(4): 667–74.

British Cohort Study (1996) *BCS70–1970 British Cohort Study Following the Lives of Everyone in Britain born 5–11 April, 1970: questionnaire used for the BCS70 fourth follow-up, 1996.* Online. Available at www.cls.ioe.ac.uk/shared/get-file.ashx?id=17&itemtype=document (accessed 28 October 2016).

Browne, A., Salmon, A. and Bassuk, S.S. (1999) 'The impact of recent partner violence on poor women's capacity to maintain work', *Violence against Women*, 5(4): 393–426.

Büsst, C. (2015a) *Alpine Health Gender Audit Focus Group Report: results from focus group discussions April 2015*, Burwood, Victoria: Deakin University.

Büsst, C. (2015b) *Murrindindi Shire Council Gender Audit Focus Group Report: results from focus group discussions June 2015*, Burwood, Victoria: Deakin University.

Chung, D., Zufferey, C. and Powell, A. (2012) *Preventing Violence against Women in the Workplace: an evidence review: full report*, Carlton, Victoria: Victorian Health Promotion Foundation.

Cunradi, C.B., Ames, G.M. and Moore, R.S. (2008) 'Prevalence and correlates of intimate partner violence among a sample of construction industry workers', *Journal of Family Violence*, 23(2): 101–12.

Dyson, S. and Flood, M. (2008) *Building Cultures of Respect and Non-Violence: a review of literature concerning adult learning and violence prevention programs with men*, Carlton, Victoria: AFL Respect and Responsibility Program and Victorian Health Promotion Foundation.

Ely, R. and Meyerson, D. (2010) 'An organizational approach to undoing gender: the unlikely case of offshore oil platforms', *Research in Organizational Behaviour*, 30: 3–34.

Fleming, P.J., Gruskin, S., Rojo, F. and Dworkin, S.L. (2015) 'Men's violence against women and men are inter-related: recommendations for simultaneous intervention', *Social Science and Medicine*, 146: 249–56.

Galvez, G., Mankowski, E.S., McGlade, M.S., Ruiz, M.E. and Glass, N. (2011) 'Work-related intimate partner violence among employed immigrants from Mexico', *Psychology of Men and Masculinity*, 12(3): 230–46.

Harvey, J. and Morris, P. (2010) *The Gender Audit Handbook: a tool for organizational self-assessment and transformation*, Washington, DC: Interaction.

Holmes, S. and Flood, M. (2013) *Genders at Work: exploring the role of workplace equality in preventing men's violence against women*, Sydney: White Ribbon Australia.

Kilgower, T. (2014) 'Staff perceptions of barriers and enablers to becoming involved in workplace-based initiatives to prevent men's violence against women', unpublished Master of Public Health thesis, Deakin University.

Kimmel, M.S. (1994) 'Masculinity and homophobia: fear, shame and silence in the construction of gender identity', in H. Brod and M. Kaufman (eds) *Theorizing Masculinities*, Thousand Oaks, CA: Sage.

Kugelberg, C. (2006) 'Constructing the deviant other: mothering and fathering at work', *Gender, Work and Organization*, 13(2): 152–73.

Lloyd, S. and Taluc, N. (1999) 'The effects of male violence on female employment', *Violence against Women*, 5(4): 370–92.

McGregor, K. (2009) *National Community Attitudes towards Violence against Women Survey 2009: project technical report*, Canberra: Australian Government, Australian Institute of Criminology.

Mankowski, E.S., Galvez, G., Perrin, N.A., Hanson, G.C. and Glass, N. (2013) 'Patterns of work-related intimate partner violence and job performance among abusive men', *Journal of Interpersonal Violence*, 28(5): 3041–58.

Max, W., Rice, D.P., Finkelstein, E., Bardwell, R.A. and Leadbetter, S. (2004) 'The economic toll of intimate partner violence against women in the United States', *Violence and Victims*, 19(3): 259–72.

Mighty, E.J. (1997) 'Conceptualizing family violence as a workplace issue: a framework for research and practice', *Employee Responsibilities and Rights Journal*, 10(4): 249–62.

Modderman, C. (2015a) *Alpine Health Gender Audit Survey Results, April 2015*, Alpine Health and Women's Health Goulburn North East.

Modderman, C. (2015b) *Murrindindi Council Gender Audit Survey Results, May 2015*, Murrindindi Shire Council and Women's Health Goulburn North East.

Moe, A.M. and Bell, M.P. (2004) 'Abject economics: the effects of battering and violence on women's work and employability', *Violence against Women*, 10(1): 29–55.

Murray, S. and Powell, A. (2007) 'Family violence prevention programs using workplaces as sites of intervention', *Research and Practice in Human Resource Management*, 15(2): 62–74.

Noblet, A.J. and LaMontagne, A. (2009) 'The challenges of developing, implementing and evaluating interventions' in S. Cartright and C.L. Cooper (eds) *Oxford Handbook of Organizational Well Being*, Oxford: Oxford University Press.

Our Watch, Australia's National Research Organisation for Women's Safety and Victorian Health Promotion Foundation (2015) *Change the Story: a shared framework for the primary prevention of violence against women and their children in Australia*, Melbourne: Our Watch.

PricewaterhouseCoopers (2015) *A High Price to Pay: the economic case for preventing violence against women*, Melbourne: PricewaterhouseCoopers.

Reeves, C. and O'Leary-Kelly, A. (2007) 'The effects and costs of intimate partner violence for work organizations', *Journal of Interpersonal Violence*, 22(3): 327–44.

Riger, S., Ahrens, C. and Blickenstaff, A. (2000) 'Measuring interference with employment and education reported by women with abusive partners: preliminary data', *Violence and Victims*, 15(2): 161–72.

Riger, S., Raja, S. and Camacho, J. (2002) 'The radiating impact of intimate partner violence', *Journal of Interpersonal Violence*, 17(2): 184–205.

Rothman, E.F. and Corso, P.S. (2008) 'Propensity for intimate partner abuse and workplace productivity: why employers should care', *Violence against Women*, 14(9): 1054–64.

Rothman, E.F. and Perry, M.J. (2004) 'Intimate partner abuse perpetrated by employees', *Journal of Occupational Health Psychology*, 9(3): 238–46.

Seymour, K. (2009) 'Women, gendered work and gendered violence: so much more than a job', *Gender, Work and Organization*, 16(2): 238–65.

Shepard, M. and Pence, E. (1988) 'The effect of battering on the employment status of women', *Affilia*, 3(2): 55–61.

Swanberg, J.E. (2004) 'Illuminating gendered organization assumptions: an important step in creating a family friendly organization: a case study', *Community, Work and Family*, 7(1): 3–28.

Swanberg, J.E. and Logan, T.K. (2005) 'Domestic violence and employment: a qualitative study', *Journal of Occupational Health Psychology*, 10(1): 3–17.

Swanberg, J.E., Logan, T.K. and Macke, C. (2005) 'Intimate partner violence, employment, and the workplace: consequences and future directions', *Trauma, Violence and Abuse*, 6(4): 286–312.

Swanberg J.E., Macke C. and Logan, T.K. (2006) 'Intimate partner violence, women and work: coping on the job', *Violence and Victims*, 21(5): 561–78.

Swanberg, J.E., Ojha, M.U. and Macke, C. (2012) 'State employment protection statutes for victims of domestic violence: public policy's response to domestic violence and an employment matter', *Journal of Interpersonal Violence*, 27(3): 587–619.

Taket, A., Turnbull, B. and Crisp, B. (2016) *Women's Health Goulburn North East Community Crime Prevention Plan – Regional Preventing Violence against Women and Children Strategy Summative Evaluation: report from the external evaluator*, February 2016. Burwood, Victoria: Deakin University.

Upston, B. and Durey, R. (2012) *Everyone's Business: a guide to developing workplace programs for the primary prevention of violence against women*, Melbourne: Women's Health Victoria.

Versola-Russo, J. and Russo F. (2009) 'When domestic violence turns into workplace violence: organizational impact and response', *Journal of Police Crisis Negotiations*, 9(2): 141–8.

VicHealth (2007) *Preventing Violence before it Occurs: a framework and background paper to guide the primary prevention of violence against women in Victoria*, Carlton, Victoria: Victorian Health Promotion Foundation.

VicHealth (2013) *Creating Healthy Workplaces: early insights from VicHealth pilot projects*, Carlton, Victoria: Victorian Health Promotion Foundation.

Wall, L. (2014) *Gender Equality and Violence against Women: what's the connection?* Canberra: Australian Institute of Family Studies.

Walters, J.L.H., Pollack, K.M., Clinton-Sherrod, M., Lindquist, C.H., McKay, T. and Lasater, B.M. (2012) 'Approaches used by employee assistance programs to address perpetration of intimate partner violence', *Violence and Victims*, 27(2): 135–47.

Wathen, C.N., MacGregor, J.C.D. and MacQuarrie, B.J. (2016) 'Relationships among intimate partner violence, work and health', *Journal of Interpersonal Violence*. Doi: 10.1177/0886260515624236.

Webster, K., Pennay, P., Bricknall, R., Diemer, K., Flood, M., Powell, A., Politoff, V. and Ward, A. (2014) *Appendixes. Australians' Attitudes to Violence against Women: findings from the 2013 National Community Attitudes towards Violence against Women Survey (NCAS)*, Melbourne: Victorian Health Promotion Foundation.

WHO (2010) *Healthy Workplaces. A Model for Action: for employers, workers, policy-makers and practitioners*, Geneva: World Health Organization.

12

POWER, PROGRESS AND PINK PUSSY HATS

Rising resistance

Ann Taket and Beth R. Crisp

Welcome to the backlash

Re-visiting a very early draft of this chapter in the cold light of early 2017 prompted reflection on earlier optimism about positive change in policy and practice, and a growing evidence base on what works in terms of eliminating gender-based violence. The election of Donald Trump in the US, despite his deeply offensive attitude towards women, and the decriminalisation of domestic violence in Russia give rise to very real concerns for the future agenda of eliminating gender-based violence. Furthermore, the worrying signs of the rise to power of the far right elected on the back of streams of untruths, insufficiently countered by fact-checking and reporting within the media, suggest that hard-won struggles for women's rights in many countries may soon be, if not already, under threat.

Claims that we must accept and inhabit a post-truth world where the untruths peddled by those in positions of power are allowed to rule must and can be resisted. The behaviour of Trump in his first weeks in office in pushing through executive orders slashing funding for a wide variety of hard-won women's health services must be seen as the resistance of patriarchal power elites to the progress won over past decades. We can take some heart from the flowering of multiple forms of resistance, making it even more imperative to continue work to develop the evidence base discussed in this book and to put it into widespread practice.

As multiple reviews (e.g. Edstrom et al. 2015; Moosa 2012) and analyses of time series data (e.g. Chon 2013; Whaley et al. 2013) have emphasised, programmes that aim to change the boundaries and expectations of what women and men can or 'should' do are often met by varying degrees of resistance; this is often referred to as 'backlash'. Recent events illustrate that this can have an extreme effect when the resistance is located in those in particular positions of power.

In what follows, we firstly summarise the types of effective approaches that can be woven together into a comprehensive programme to prevent gender-based violence. The chapter then considers some of the key challenges and issues before moving on to address the response in terms of the rise in resistance to the backlash we have noted above. The chapter concludes with a consideration of what will be needed to retain the elimination of gender-based violence on the policy and practice agendas.

The need for a multi-faceted approach

As we emphasised in Chapter 1, a simplistic understanding of the factors resulting in gender-based violence will lead to ineffective policy and programme responses. Rather, action is required in all sectors of society to address the economic, political and social structures that subordinate women, based on an intersectional analysis that recognises the other factors that are also at play. *Change the Story* (Our Watch et al. 2015a, 2015b), the framework for primary prevention in Australia, discussed this in terms of five essential and five supporting actions (Table 12.1) that require legislative, institutional and policy responses. Settings for specific programmes of action that need to be involved include educational institutions (at all levels from kindergarten to university and vocational education), workplaces, sports clubs and other community settings, media and popular culture.

Ellsberg et al. (2015) in their review classified interventions by the broad strategy adopted and conclude that there are four approaches with promising evidence: economic empowerment or income supplementation combined with gender equality training; empowerment training to improve the agency of women; workshops to

TABLE 12.1 Key actions to prevent GBV

Essential actions to address the gendered drivers of violence	*Supporting actions to address reinforcing factors*
Challenge condoning of violence against women	Challenge the normalisation of violence as an expression of masculinity or male dominance
Promote women's independence and decision-making in public life and relationships	Prevent exposure to violence and support those affected to reduce its consequences
Foster positive personal identities and challenge gender stereotypes and roles	Address the intersections between social norms relating to alcohol and gender
Strengthen positive, equal and respectful relations between people of all ages and genders	Reduce backlash by engaging men and boys in gender equality, building relationship skills and social connections
Promote and normalise gender equality in public and private life	Promote broader social equality and address structural discrimination and disadvantage

Source: Adapted from Our Watch et al. 2015a: 13.

address gender and behavioural norms among men and women; and participatory or community-driven development. Examples of each of these have appeared in the earlier chapters of this book. The Ellsberg et al. review was based on what they call 'rigorously evaluated studies' that measured impact on at least one specific type of violence against women and girls. They note that some of the areas where they found insufficient evidence could well have resulted from underpowered studies rather than a definite absence of effect (Ellsberg et al. 2015: 1564).

Michau et al. (2015) consider a much wider range of research as well as practice experience in their review paper, to identify five core principles that need to inform programming to prevent gender-based violence:

> first, analysis and actions to prevent violence across the social ecology . . .; second, intervention designs based on an intersectional gender-power analysis; third, theory-informed models developed on the basis of evidence; fourth, sustained investment in multisector interventions; and finally, aspirational programming that promotes personal and collective thought, and enables activism.
>
> *(Michau et al. 2015: 1672)*

As Chapter 1 emphasised, it is important that programming is gender transformative, and sustained advocacy by women's movements at all levels is vital. Examples of such programming have been discussed throughout the book. Garcia-Moreno et al. (2015) present a call to action at the conclusion to *The Lancet* series of papers of which Ellsberg et al. (2015) and Michau et al. (2015) are part; this emphasises the political leadership and governmental investment that is required.

Looking back over the earlier chapters, in Chapter 1, the section on gender mainstreaming illustrated work at the global level and demonstrated the importance of strong transnational advocacy networks, in particular the transnational feminist movement, in the positive results achieved. We also saw how intersectionality is increasingly being recognised in terms of guidance at the global level (for example, Stephens et al. 2017). The section on economic empowerment in Chapter 1 illustrated examples at both global and societal levels. At the societal level, examples of successful initiatives for economic empowerment in a variety of low- and middle-income countries were discussed, and the importance of the influence of global institutions such as the World Bank and UNDP was also examined.

Chapter 1 also explored an example of a very successful community mobilisation initiative, presented as a case study owing to its rigorous evaluation through randomised control trial and an embedded qualitative research component. Illustrations of successful community mobilisation were covered in some of the work presented in Chapter 8 on engaging bystanders in violence prevention.

Successful initiatives in different settings have been illustrated throughout the book, some chapters being focused on a single setting, others illustrating programmes that have been used in multiple settings. Chapter 2, in discussing work with parents and young families, included work in antenatal care, maternal and child health, and community settings. Schools, a particularly important setting, were the focus of Chapters 3, 4 and 5 and were also covered in Chapter 8. Chapter 3 covered respectful relationships education, emphasising the importance of this being taken on from a whole-school perspective, while Chapters 4, 5 and 8 focused on different programmes (*Green Acres High, You the Man*) which could form part of a whole-school approach to respectful relationships education. Colleges and universities were the focus for Chapter 6, with an emphasis on a system-wide, whole-of-institution perspective; universities were also covered in Chapters 7 and 8 which focused on different programmes (ESD, *You the Man*) which could form a part of a whole-institution approach.

Chapters 9, 10 and 11 each focused on a different setting. Chapter 9 considered faith communities as a setting for violence prevention, covering some particular initiatives and identifying their limitations, illustrating that although a setting with much potential, this has still to be fully realised. Chapter 10 then considered health and social care as a setting, identifying the scope in professional practice and the setting environment for supporting primary prevention, while also discussing some of the challenges that remain to be overcome. Chapter 11 focused on workplaces as a setting, reviewing the importance of the prevention of gender-based violence to employers in terms of effects on business efficiency as well as in terms of importance in terms of prevention, and explored an asset-based approach that is being used in two workplaces in rural Victoria.

Challenges and issues

Avoiding harmful effects

Safety is an important consideration in providing any programme, service or research aimed at informing programme design or evaluating programme effectiveness. This is particularly so when the topic concerned is that of interpersonal violence. The manual produced by Ellsberg and Heise (2005) discusses the methodological and ethical challenges of conducting research on violence against women and describes a range of ways to tackle these challenges, drawing on the collective experience of researchers and activists. These ideas are just as applicable in the design of prevention programmes.

Fleming et al. (2014) illustrates the importance of adopting gender-transformative interventions that challenge harmful hegemonic masculine norms using the example of the inadvertent harmful effects of *Man Up Monday*, a media campaign to prevent the spread of sexually transmitted infections. Müller and Shahrokh (2016) summarise findings from programmes that focus on structural and institutional factors in a variety of countries: Egypt, India, Kenya, Sierra Leone, South Africa and Uganda. They conclude by emphasising the importance of moving beyond male protectionism and paternalism:

Where work with men is building on men's concern for women's safety, as in work with men to address SGBV [sexual and gender-based violence], risks of strengthening patriarchal norms are high. Engaging men should not reinforce a sense of male supremacy, by simply appealing to men as 'protectors' of women and girls. Men should be engaged as agents of change holding themselves and their communities accountable for rejecting SGBV on the grounds of dismantling oppression and claiming human rights. Working together with women to challenge problematic gender roles and expectations amongst both men and women strengthens this accountability and provides space for mutual learning and redefinition of harmful gender norms.

(*Müller and Shahrokh 2016: 4*)

The importance of a carefully constructed comprehensive and intersectional approach is also illustrated by the work of Rahman (2016). Rahman examines the discursive construction of 'culture' and 'social norms' in well-intentioned documents – such as the *United Nations General Recommendation No. 19* on violence against women (which brought violence against women within the realm of international human rights law), special rapporteurs' reports relevant to the *Convention on the Elimination of All Forms of Discrimination against Women* (CEDAW), country reports, *World Report on Violence and Health* and research literature on male IPV (intimate partner violence) against women in Bangladesh. Although these documents were intended to negate 'harmful cultural practices' and eliminate 'all forms of discrimination against women', Rahman's analysis shows that they have in contrast been appropriating colonial/neocolonial and patriarchal structures and, in turn, contributing to othering the women living in the Global South including Bangladesh.

Engaging men

Another major challenge that we have noted in various places throughout the book is that of engaging men. Berkowitz (2001, 2004), writing specifically about the prevention of sexual assault, finds that effective programmes offer positive messages which build on men's values and predisposition to act in a positive manner. This was very much the approach adopted in the design of *You the Man*, discussed in Chapter 8, where the play serves to introduce the participants to a variety of positive male role models in relation to sexual assault and dating violence in a way that engages cognitive, affective and behavioural domains: what people know, how they feel and how they behave (another of Berkowitz's elements of effective programmes). *Bell Bajao!* and *Soul City*, also discussed in Chapter 8, are designed similarly.

Also important is the so-called 'teachable moment' (Lewis 1982; Nutting 1986), a moment or even period when life circumstances are such that people are particularly receptive to new knowledge, reflecting on attitudes held and consideration of behaviour change. One such teachable moment is during the transition to parenthood. Programmes like *Baby Makes 3*, discussed in Chapter 2, are explicitly designed to target this teachable period, a time when parents–to-be often seek out information to prepare for and respond to the arrival of a new family member. This is echoed in the analysis offered by Casey et al. (2013) who examined the challenges of engaging men based on interviews with representatives of 29 organisations engaging men and boys in preventing violence against women in Africa, Asia, Europe, Oceania, and North and South America. They identify the importance of strengths-based outreach that approaches men as partners in prevention, and of initiating conversations on issues of central importance to men, such as fatherhood and relationships.

Other initiatives draw attention to the high cost for men of maintaining patriarchal privileges in terms of compromised physical and mental health, heightened risk for injury, limited intimacy and superficial friendships (Messner 1997; Morrell et al. 2012). Dworkin et al. (2013) provide an example of one programme, *One Man Can*, a rights-based gender equality and health programme implemented by Sonke Gender Justice in South Africa; their results indicate that the programme has shifted men's attitudes about gender roles and power relations in the direction of gender equality, and improved numerous health outcomes, due to reduced alcohol use, safer sex and reductions in male violence, against both women and men (van den Berg et al. 2013). Viitanen and Colvin (2015) researched *One Man Can*, alongside other gender and health intervention programmes in South Africa, looking at how the men participating in these programmes responded to three thematic messages often found in gender transformative work: the 'costs of masculinity' men pay for adherence to harmful gender constructs; multiple forms of masculinity; and a human rights framework and contested rights. Overall the men were receptive to the messages and could relate them to the contexts of their own lives; however, some men were more ambivalent to shifting gender norms and discussions over gender equity.

These provide just some specific examples of progress being made in tackling the challenge of engaging men. The range of successful programmes that involve work with men and boys to change attitudes, behaviours and social norms is diverse and growing (Barker et al. 2007; IPPF 2010; Jewkes et al. 2015); the challenge remaining is to ensure that this growth continues and that these programmes are developed in a synergistic rather than siloed way (Michau et al. 2015).

Resisting the tyranny of evidence hierarchies

Throughout this book a wide variety of different types of evidence has been used, drawing on many different disciplines, including political science, sociology and anthropology as well as the disciplines more familiar to public health researchers. The use of all these different types of evidence is important, and they need to be valued for the insight and contribution they can all provide. Once we are researching the operation of system-wide strategies that bring together multiple actors in their implementation, the simple hierarchy of evidence (Guyatt et al. 2000) that considers a number of randomised control trials as the gold standard becomes irrelevant (Petticrew and Roberts 2003). A randomised control trial to 'prove' the insights we have gained as to the importance of strong advocacy networks in progress on gender mainstreaming (as discussed in Chapter 1), for example, could not even be designed, let alone carried out.

A much more helpful approach to summarising what is known about particular types of programme is that described and used in Barker et al. (2007) (see Figure 12.1). This is particularly important for its recognition of the value of qualitative research as on a par with quantitative research.

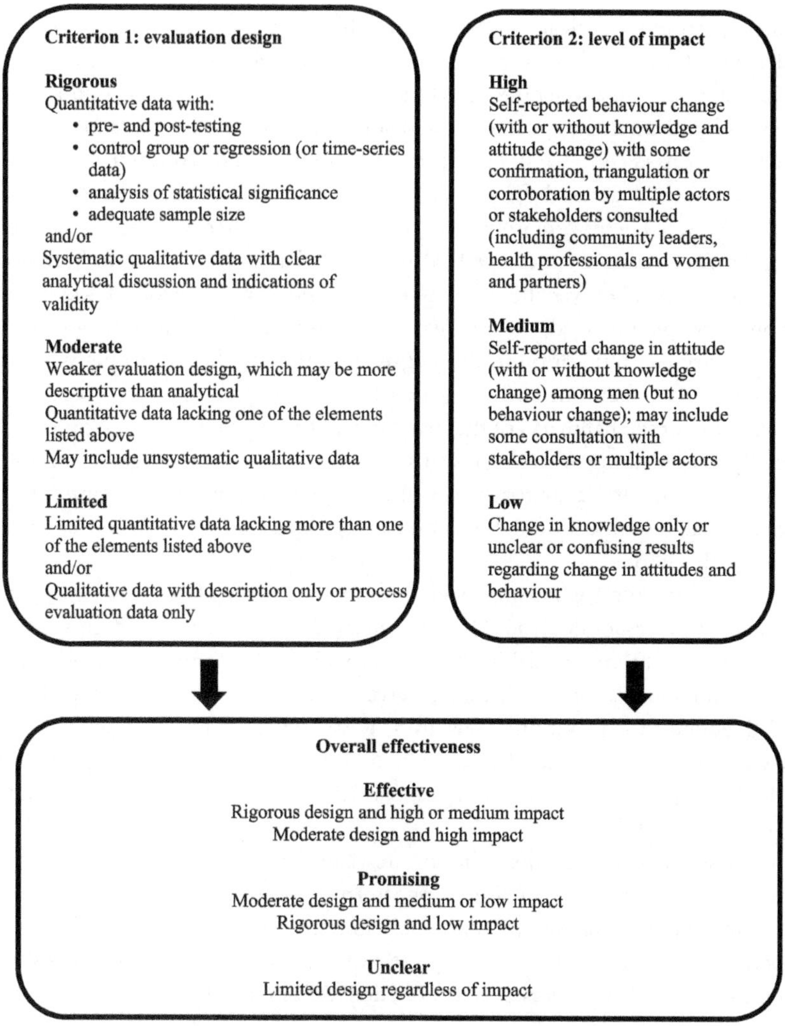

Criterion 1: evaluation design

Rigorous
Quantitative data with:
- pre- and post-testing
- control group or regression (or time-series data)
- analysis of statistical significance
- adequate sample size
and/or
Systematic qualitative data with clear analytical discussion and indications of validity

Moderate
Weaker evaluation design, which may be more descriptive than analytical
Quantitative data lacking one of the elements listed above
May include unsystematic qualitative data

Limited
Limited quantitative data lacking more than one of the elements listed above
and/or
Qualitative data with description only or process evaluation data only

Criterion 2: level of impact

High
Self-reported behaviour change (with or without knowledge and attitude change) with some confirmation, triangulation or corroboration by multiple actors or stakeholders consulted (including community leaders, health professionals and women and partners)

Medium
Self-reported change in attitude (with or without knowledge change) among men (but no behaviour change); may include some consultation with stakeholders or multiple actors

Low
Change in knowledge only or unclear or confusing results regarding change in attitudes and behaviour

Overall effectiveness

Effective
Rigorous design and high or medium impact
Moderate design and high impact

Promising
Moderate design and medium or low impact
Rigorous design and low impact

Unclear
Limited design regardless of impact

FIGURE 12.1 Examining programme effectiveness – use of evidence

Source: Adapted from Barker et al. (2007: 13).

Very importantly, resisting the tyranny of evidence hierarchies does not amount to discarding research evidence in favour of so-called alternative truths. All types of research evidence have their role to play in countering the alternative truths foisted upon us by those who see their power and privilege as threatened. Nevertheless, research evidence should lead to action. As such, 'we believe evidence-based practice and research cannot and must not replace participation in broad-based activism to confront inequalities and injustice' (Beddoe and Maidment 2009: 134).

Remaining positive

While supportive political will was definitely not evident in early 2017 in the leadership of two of the most significant countries globally, namely the US and Russia, there are very welcome signs of an increased level of resistance in response. Advocates and international NGOs and social movements have ensured that the backlash that has been seen has not gone uncontested. Anti-Trump marches round the world were organised for the day after the inauguration of the 45th president of the US. These were impressive in bringing together support for the whole range of intersectional issues involved in gender-based violence. What impressed us about the marches was the diversity of men and women involved, the number of young people involved, the absence of the traditional organisations of the left, the creativity and innovation in the slogans, and the number of people who were marching for the first time and seeing that act as the beginning of a whole series of actions. One of the hallmarks of the marches was the appearance of pink pussy hats, carefully crafted along with slogans to show resistance to the offensive comments Trump made about his approach to women. Other slogans drew attention to the intersectional response required, and we have selected just some of these as a fitting cover for this book.

But the response has not just been by non-state actors. Governments in other countries have responded too. On 23 January 2017, Trump signed an executive order banning international NGOs from providing abortion services or offering information about abortions if they receive US funding, the so-called 'global gag rule' (Redden 2017). Within a few days it was reported by the Dutch international development minister that up to 20 countries have indicated support for the Netherlands' plan to set up an international safe abortion fund to plug the funding gap (Darroch 2017).

It is also important to note that the resistance is not just seen in one day of marches; we have also seen a rise in long-term responses and sharing of resources for use in supporting action. Within the US in response to the election of Trump, an all-volunteer group of 'like-minded professional activists, students and artists' have come together as '1460 Days of Action'. Their website clarifies:

> Our mission: 1460 is dedicated to promoting democratic values in America and supporting candidates committed to them.

Our vision is a nation where all people are represented by an inclusive government that reflects America's broad diversity.

(1460 Days of Action 2017)

The 1460 Days of Action website also provides suggested actions for every day and a toolkit for change, containing knowledge about rights, how to lobby elected representatives, organisations working to stand up for individuals being harassed, and initiatives like 'Solidarity Sundays', a nationwide network of feminist activist groups.

Other websites such as Hollaback! emphasise particular types of action. Hollaback! is a global movement which describes its work as being:

Our mission is to build safe, inclusive public spaces by transforming the culture that perpetuates discrimination and violence.

We carry out this mission by building the power of people to create measurable and long-lasting impacts in the movement for gender justice.

(Hollaback! n.d.)

The Hollaback! website provides a wide range of resources including safety guides and bystander training.

There are examples to be found at all ecological levels; see for example Michau et al. (2015). While an exhaustive review is impossible, at the other end of the spectrum from the above initiatives, which are global or international in scope, we present just two examples of very local-level initiatives near to where we are located, led by men, which address GBV. First of all, MENd: an initiative run within a suburb of Melbourne which uses Facebook 'So men (and women) can learn about the impacts of Gender Inequity. So men can be part of the culture that changes attitudes' (MENd n.d.). The second example, on a slightly larger scale, is the Man Cave, which also utilises Facebook for communicating its message: 'Deconstruct | Challenge | Redefine: A preventative mental health and emotional intelligence program for boys & young men.' As its website explains, Man Cave (n.d.) has been operating since 2014, and as Jacks (2015) explains, it links what it does directly to preventing violence against women.

All of the above are encouraging as examples of action and community mobilisation or citizen engagement that is strongly rooted in protecting and defending human rights and working towards equality. Writing in a rather different context, but of particular interest in terms of its global coverage, Gaventa and Barrett (2010) explored the outcomes of citizen engagement through a systematic meta-analysis of 100 researched case studies of citizen engagement in 20 different countries; most of the cases were from low- and middle-income countries. Some, but not all, of these dealt specifically with gender-based violence. They examined four different types of outcome: construction of citizenship, including both knowledge and sense of agency and empowerment; strengthening practices of participation;

strengthening the responsiveness and accountability of states; and finally developing inclusive and cohesive societies. They found positive outcomes in relation to each of these different types, although not uniformly across all cases, the overall ratio of positive to negative outcomes being 3 to 1. Their findings point to the relative importance of associations and social movements compared with institutionalised fora for participatory governance, and to the need for multiple strategies of engagement. Interestingly no simple linear relationship between level of democratisation and level of positive outcomes was found; instead the highest incidence of positive outcomes are in the weakest and most fragile democracies, many of which are characterised by recent histories of conflict or violence.

Future work

First and foremost in terms of future work is the need for continued activism at all levels to resist the backlash currently seen in the US, UK, Australia and Europe. Here it is particularly important to foster advocacy and social movements and their international linkage. Programmes and advocacy at all levels need to recognise intersectionality and the necessity for work on all human rights issues. In particular we would emphasise the usefulness of a human rights grounding for intersectional practice.

While continuing to advocate for the significant levels of funding necessary for eliminating GBV, it is also important to defend funding for the necessary levels of response services to address the needs of those who have experienced gender-based violence as well as those who perpetrate it. Funding for the elimination of GBV cannot substitute for funding response services in the short or medium term, only in the longer term when further progress has been made towards the goal of eliminating GBV.

In designing programmes for primary prevention, it is important to recognise the value of different types of research evidence including that produced by communities of practice, and to ensure that programmes have a clear theory of change underlying them. We also need to recognise that insufficient evaluation has been carried out in many cases, often due to lack of appropriate levels of funding, and seek to rectify this in future.

We dedicated this volume to all those who dare to believe, and dare to act, to eliminate gender-based violence, and to other human rights defenders everywhere. Efforts at both gaining and maintaining policy and practice vistas which support the elimination of gender-based violence are going to continue to be required into the foreseeable future, and probably for much longer than 1,460 days. While short-term acts of resistance can be vital in placing gender-based violence in public purview, strategies for sustaining this work in the long term will be essential. At an individual level, this includes 'courage to make relationships with people who are distressed, ability to face anger and grief, perseverance in the face of disappointment, and ability to maintain respect' (Beddoe and Maidment 2009: 133). For organisations, this will involve not only providing support to front-line workers, but an organisational culture in which good practice includes time for reflection and where failure to succeed is recognised as an opportunity to explore new ways of thinking and working rather than a reason to cease this often difficult work (Hawkins and Shohet 2012). Finally, as we emphasised earlier, continued advocacy by internationally linked feminist and pro-feminist networks will continue to be essential.

References

1460 Days of Action (2017) 'What is 1460 Days of Action?' Online. Available at www.1460. live/what-is-1460-days-of-action/ (accessed 28 March 2017).

Barker, G., Ricardo, C. and Nascimento, M. (2007) *Engaging Men and Boys in Changing Gender-Based Inequity in Health: evidence from programme interventions*, Geneva: World Health Organization.

Beddoe, L. and Maidment, J. (2009) *Mapping Knowledge for Social Work Practice: critical intersections*, South Melbourne: Cengage Learning.

Berkowitz, A.D. (2001) 'Critical elements of sexual assault prevention and risk reduction programs', in C. Kilmartin (ed.) *Sexual Assault in Context: teaching college men about gender*, Holmes Beach, FL: Learning Publications.

Berkowitz, A.D. (2004) *The Social Norms Approach: theory, research and annotated bibliography*. Online. Available at www.alanberkowitz.com/articles/social_norms.pdf (accessed 23 March 2016).

Casey, E.A., Carlson, J., Fraguela-Rios, C., Kimball, E., Neugut, T.B., Tolman, R.M. and Edleson, J.L. (2013) 'Context, challenges, and tensions in global efforts to engage men in the prevention of violence against women: an ecological analysis', *Men and Masculinities*, 16: 228–51.

Chon, D.S. (2013) 'Test of impacts of gender equality and economic development on sexual violence', *Journal of Family Violence*, 28: 603–10.

Darroch, G. (2017) 'Dutch respond to Trump's "gag rule" with international safe abortion fund', *The Guardian*. Online. Available at www.theguardian.com/global-development/2017/jan/25/netherlands-trump-gag-rule-international-safe-abortion-fund (accessed 12 March 2017).

Dworkin, S.L., Hatcher, A.M., Colvin, C. and Peacock, D. (2013) 'Impact of a gender-transformative HIV and antiviolence programme on gender ideologies and masculinities in two rural, South African communities', *Men and Masculinities*, 16: 181–202.

Edstrom, J., Hassink, A., Shahrokh, T. and Stern, E. (2015) *Engendering Men: a collaborative review of evidence on men and boys in social change and gender equality*, Brighton: Promundo-US, Sonke Gender Justice and the Institute of Development Studies.

Ellsberg, M. and Heise, L. (2005) *Researching Violence against Women: a practical guide or researchers and activists*, Washington, DC: World Health Organization, PATH.

Ellsberg, M., Arango, D.J., Morton, M., Gennari, F., Kiplesund, S., Contreras, M. and Watts, C. (2015) 'Prevention of violence against women and girls: what does the evidence say?' *The Lancet*, 385: 1555–66.

Fleming, P.J., Lee, J.G.L. and Dworkin, S.L. (2014) '"Real men don't": constructions of masculinity and inadvertent harm in public health interventions', *American Journal of Public Health*, 104: 1029–35.

García-Moreno, C., Zimmerman, C., Morris-Gehring, A., Heise, L., Amin, A., Abrahams, N., Montoya, O., Bhate-Deosthali, P., Kilonzo, N. and Watts, C. (2015) 'Addressing violence against women: a call to action', *The Lancet*, 385: 1685–95.

Gaventa, J. and Barrett, G. (2010) *So What Difference Does It Make? Mapping the outcomes of citizen engagement*, Brighton: Institute of Development Studies, IDS Working Paper 347.

Guyatt, G.H., Haynes, R.B., Jaeschke, R.Z., Cook, D.J., Green, L., Naylor, C.D., Wilson, M.C. and Richardson W.S. (2000) 'Users' guides to the medical literature: XXV. Evidence-based medicine: principles for applying the users' guides to patient care', *Journal of the American Medical Association*, 284: 1290–6.

Hawkins, P. and Shohet, R. (2012) *Supervision in the Helping Professions*, 4th edn, Maidenhead: Open University Press.

Hollaback! (n.d.) *About Hollaback!*. Online. Available at www.ihollaback.org/about/ (accessed 28 March 2017).

IPPF (2010) *Men are Changing: case study evidence on work with men and boys to promote gender equality and positive masculinities*, London: International Planned Parenthood Federation.

Jacks, T. (2015) 'From boys to men', *The Age*, 30 May 2015.

Jewkes, R., Flood, M. and Lang, J. (2015) 'From work with men and boys to changes of social norms and reduction of inequities in gender relations: a conceptual shift in prevention of violence against women and girls', *The Lancet*, 385: 1580–9.

Lewis, C.E. (1982) 'Teaching medical students about disease prevention and health promotion', *Public Health Reports*, 97: 210–15.

Man Cave (n.d.) *The Man Cave*. Online. Available at www.facebook.com/themancaveAU (accessed 28 March 2017).

MENd (n.d.) *Gender Equality is not a Women's Issue*. Online. Available at www.facebook.com/ MENdEquality (accessed 28 March 2017).

Messner, M.A. (1997) *Politics of Masculinities: men in movements*, Thousand Oaks, CA: Sage.

Michau, L., Horn, J., Bank, A., Dutt, M. and Zimmerman, C. (2015) 'Prevention of violence against women and girls: lessons from practice', *The Lancet*, 385: 1672–84.

Moosa, Z. (2012) *A Theory of Change for Tackling Violence against Women and Girls*, London: ActionAid.

Morrell, R., Jewkes, R. and Lindegger, G. (2012) 'Hegemonic masculinity/masculinities in South Africa: culture, power, and gender politics', *Men and Masculinities*, 15: 11–30.

Müller, C. and Shahrokh, T. (2016) *Engaging Men for Effective Activism against Sexual and Gender-Based Violence*, Brighton: Institute of Development Studies.

Nutting, P.A. (1986) 'Health promotion in primary medical care: problems and potential', *Preventive Medicine*, 15(5): 537–48.

Our Watch, Australia's National Research Organisation for Women's Safety and Victorian Health Promotion Foundation (2015a) *Change the Story: a shared framework for the primary prevention of violence against women and their children in Australia*, Melbourne: Our Watch.

Our Watch, Australia's National Research Organisation for Women's Safety and VicHealth (2015b) *Framework Foundations 1: a review of the evidence on correlates of violence against women and what works to prevent it. Companion document to Change the Story: a shared framework for the primary prevention of violence against women and their children in Australia*, Melbourne: Our Watch.

Petticrew, M. and Roberts, H. (2003) 'Evidence, hierarchies, and typologies: horses for courses', *Journal of Epidemiology and Community Health*, 57: 527–9.

Rahman, L. (2016) Othering the post-colonial women in 'harmful cultural practices' and 'social norms' discourses in addressing the male intimate partner violence in Bangladesh. Seminar presented at Munk School of Global Affairs, University of Toronto.

Redden, M. (2017) '"Global gag rule" reinstated by Trump, curbing NGO abortion services abroad', *The Guardian*. Online. Available at www.theguardian.com/world/2017/jan/23/trump-abortion-gag-rule-international-ngo-funding (accessed 12 March 2017).

Stephens, A., Lewis, E.D. and Reddy, S. (2017) *Inclusive Systemic Evaluation for Gender Equality, Goals, Environments, and Voices from the Margins (ISE4GEMs): a guidance for evaluators for the SDG Era*, New York: UN Women.

van den Berg, W., Hendricks, L., Hatcher, A., Peacock, D., Godana, P. and Dworkin, S. (2013) '*One Man Can*: shifts in fatherhood beliefs and parenting practices following a gender-transformative programme in Eastern Cape, South Africa', *Gender and Development*, 21: 111–25.

Viitanen, A.P. and Colvin, C.J. (2015) 'Lessons learned: program messaging in gender-transformative work with men and boys in South Africa', *Global Health Action*, 8: 27860. Online. Available at http://dx.doi.org/10.3402/gha.v8.27860 (accessed 5 February 2016).

Whaley, R.B., Messner, S.F. and Veysey, B.M. (2013) 'The relationship between gender equality and rates of inter- and intra-sexual lethal violence: an exploration of functional form', *Justice Quarterly*, 30: 732–54.

INDEX

Page numbers in *italic* relate to figures, page numbers in **bold** relate to tables.